PRACTICAL SOCIAL WORK

Series Editor: Jo Campling

BASW

Editorial Advisory Board:
Robert Adams, Terry Bamford, Charles Barker, Lena Dominelli,
Malcolm Payne, Michael Preston-Shoot, Daphne Statham and
Jane Tunstill

Social work is at an important stage in its development. All professions must be responsive to changing social and economic conditions if they are to meet the needs of those they serve. This series focuses on sound practice and the specific contribution which social workers can make to the well-being of our society in the 1990s.

The British Association of Social Workers has always been conscious of its role in setting guidelines for practice and in seeking to raise professional standards. The conception of the Practical Social Work series arose from a survey of BASW members to discover where they, the practitioners in social work, felt there was the most need for new literature. The response was overwhelming and enthusiastic, and the result is a carefully planned, coherent series of books. The emphasis is firmly on practice, set in a theoretical framework. The books will inform, stimulate and promote discussion, thus adding to the further development of skills and high professional standards. All the authors are practitioners and teachers of social work, representing a wide variety of experience.

JO CAMPLING

A list of published titles in this series follows overleaf

PRACTICAL SOCIAL WORK

PUBLISHED

Robert Adams *Self-Help, Social Work and Empowerment*

David Anderson *Social Work and Mental Handicap*

James G. Barber *Beyond Casework*

Peter Beresford and Suzy Croft *Citizen Involvement: A Practical Guide for Change*

Suzy Braye and Michael Preston-Shoot *Practising Social Work Law*

Robert Brown, Stanley Bute and Peter Ford *Social Workers at Risk*

Alan Butler and Colin Pritchard *Social Work and Mental Illness*

Crescy Cannan, Lynne Berry and Karen Lyons *Social Work and Europe*

Roger Clough *Residential Work*

David M. Cooper and David Ball *Social Work and Child Abuse*

Veronica Coulshed *Management in Social Work*

Veronica Coulshed *Social Work Practice: An introduction (2nd edn)*

Paul Daniel and John Wheeler *Social Work and Local Politics*

Peter R. Day *Sociology in Social Work Practice*

Lena Dominelli *Anti-Racist Social Work: A Challenge for White Practitioners and Educators*

Celia Doyle *Working with Abused Children*

Angela Everitt, Pauline Hardiker, Jane Littlewood and Audrey Mullender *Applied Research for Better Practice*

Kathy Ford and Alan Jones *Student Supervision*

David Francis and Paul Henderson *Working with Rural Communities*

Michael D. A. Freeman *Children, their Families and the Law*

Alison Froggatt *Family Work with Elderly People*

Danya Glaser and Stephen Frosh *Child Sexual Abuse*

Bryan Glastonbury *Computers in Social Work*

Gill Gorell Barnes *Working with Families*

Cordelia Grimwood and Ruth Popplestone *Women, Management and Care*

Jalna Hanmer and Daphne Statham *Women and Social Work: Towards a Woman-Centred Practice*

Tony Jeffs and Mark Smith (eds) *Youth Work*

Michael Kerfoot and Alan Butler *Problems of Childhood and Adolescence*

Joyce Lishman *Communication in Social Work*

Mary Marshall *Social Work with Old People (2nd edn)*

Paula Nicolson and Rowan Bayne *Applied Psychology for Social Workers (2nd edn)*

Kieran O'Hagan *Crisis Intervention in Social Services*

Michael Oliver *Social Work with Disabled People*

Joan Orme and Bryan Glastonbury *Care Management: Tasks and Workloads*

Malcolm Payne *Social Care in the Community*

Malcolm Payne *Working in Teams*

John Pitts *Working with Young Offenders*

Michael Preston-Shoot *Effective Groupwork*

Carole R. Smith *Adoption and Fostering: Why and How*

Carole R. Smith *Social Work with the Dying and Bereaved*

Carole R. Smith, Marty T. Lane and Terry Walsh *Child Care and the Courts*

Gill Stewart and John Stewart *Social Work and Housing*

Christine Stones *Focus on Families*

Neil Thompson *Anti-Discriminatory Practice*

Neil Thompson with Michael Murphy and Steve Stradling *Dealing with Stress*

Derek Tilbury *Working with Mental Illness*

Alan Twelvetrees *Community Work (2nd edn)*

Hilary Walker and Bill Beaumount (eds) *Working with Offenders*

Applied Research for Better Practice

Angela Everitt
Pauline Hardiker
Jane Littlewood
and
Audrey Mullender

Foreword by Jo Campling

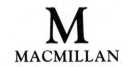

MACMILLAN

First published 1992 by
THE MACMILLAN PRESS LTD
Houndmills, Basingstoke, Hampshire RG21 2XS
and London
Companies and representatives
throughout the world

ISBN 0–333–54433–1 hardcover
ISBN 0–333–54434–X paperback

A catalogue record for this book is available from the British Library.

Reprinted 1994

Printed in Hong Kong

Series Standing Order (Practical Social Work)

If you would like to receive future titles in this series as they are published, you can make use of our standing order facility. To place a standing order please contact your bookseller or, in case of difficulty,write to us at the address below with your name and address and the name of the series. Please state with which title you wish to begin your standing order. (If you live outside the United Kingdom we may not have the rights for your area, in which case we will forward your order to the publisher concerned.)

Customer Services Department, Macmillan Distribution Ltd
Houndmills, Basingstoke, Hampshire RG21 2XS, England

Contents

Foreword

Applied Research for Better Practice is a welcome addition to the Practical Social Work series. It is not a research methods handbook or toolkit, but rather an attempt to develop a social work methodology grounded in the values, knowledge and skills required for critical inquiry and participatory methods of research.

The authors believe that 'research-mindedness' enhances good practices in social work, and that research and practice can be conceptualised as an inter-related process. Such a belief is only justified, however, if certain intellectual and professional principles are upheld. First, a participatory/developmental rather than a social control model of social work is adopted. Second, anti-oppressive values are applied. Third, practitioners strive towards a genuine model of partnership with those whom they serve. This means that clients are not treated as objects; that the bases of 'knowing' are shared and made explicit as much as possible; and that subjectivity is valued and understood in the contexts of the often vulnerable circumstances of people's lives.

Research-minded practice is explored in a holistic way in this book. Problem formulation, data collection, data analysis and evaluation are not treated as discrete stages in the supposedly linear process of research. Instead, each of these is addressed using the same framework: values, purposes, ethics, communication, roles and skills. Anti-oppressive practices and developmental principles also anchor the process from beginning to end.

The authors do not make claims for a definitive methodology for the research-minded practitioner. Rather they make some tentative approximations and provisional suggestions in what is obviously a potentially complex project. But above all, as we enter a new era in the mixed economy of welfare and criminal justice, the authors develop an approach in which the achievements of the welfare state can be reclaimed and developed even where the structural space afforded the practitioner is changing rapidly. This will only be possible if the values, knowledge and skills underlying the appraisal adopted in this book are developed in the interests of 'applied research for better practice'.

JO CAMPLING

Acknowledgements

Our ideas for this book have developed through valuable discussions with colleagues, students and practitioners. We have benefited from many who have listened to us, challenged and informed our thinking about research-mindedness in social work and tested out our ideas in practice. In particular, we express our appreciation to those associated with the Social Welfare Research Unit at Newcastle Polytechnic, the School of Social Work at the University of Leicester, the Department of Social Sciences at Loughborough University, and the Centre for Applied Social Studies at the University of Durham.

The value base in Chapter 3 draws on the groupwork research conducted and written up elsewhere jointly by Audrey Mullender and Dave Ward. We also acknowledge the work of students on the 1989–91 MA Social Work course at the University of Leicester. Their work in a research methods workshop generated many of the examples used in Chapter 5.

Dorothy Stock Whittaker has done much to encourage practitioners to undertake research. She has taken a lively interest in our work and offered wise advice and guidance. Jo Campling helped us get started and encouraged us along the way. Pam Carter has been invaluable as our unofficial editor. We thank them all.

Language is powerful. It is not neutral. In this book we make the point that language must continuously be examined for the part it may play in discriminatory and oppressive mechanisms. We have tried to do this in our own writing. However, in the interests of accuracy, material from other authors has been left in its original form. Sometimes our own language, and that of others, will be experienced as oppressive. For this we apologise.

ANGELA EVERITT
PAULINE HARDIKER
JANE LITTLEWOOD
AUDREY MULLENDER

1

Research and Practice

In this book we address the relationship between research and social work by exploring the possibilities of integrating research with practice. This is not a research methods text. Our intention is not to provide advice and guidance to enable social workers to undertake research or even to implement the findings from research into their practice. Rather our aim is to learn from research methodology and methods so as to contribute to the development of social work methodology and methods: to develop a social work practice informed by and infused with understanding of research methodology and methods: to provide a methodology for the research-minded practitioner; to develop a critical, reflective practice.

The relationship between research and social work is problematic. Government committee reports (Younghusband, 1959; Seebohm, 1968), writers (Holman, 1970; Shaw, 1975; Carew, 1979; Kahan, 1989) and working parties established to address the issue (Pinker, 1978; CCETSW/PSSC, 1980) have acknowledged this. Attention has been drawn to social workers not pursuing research, not implementing the findings of research in their practice, nor even reading research reports. Sinfield criticised the Seebohm Committee for failing to undertake research. He pointed out that, despite having powers to do so, both central and local government had done little to encourage and initiate research in social work (Sinfield, 1969). The knowledge base of social work has been described as one of pragmatism or, at best, practice wisdom. Social workers have little time for systematically analysing social need and inequality, social policies and resources, to inform practice. For their part, social workers have criticised researchers for being detached, elitist and preaching about practice from a distance (Cohen, 1975). Social work practitioners and activists, sometimes

1

supported by social theorists, have expressed frustration with research and theory for failing to have an impact on the pursuit of justice (Deutsch and Howard, 1970; Gouldner, 1971). And yet there is a lost tradition of research in social work which we will explore later in this introductory chapter.

In this chapter we introduce the idea of the research-minded practitioner. We examine possible reasons for practitioners being alienated from research and explore recent programmes and initiatives which may have had the effect of bringing research and social work closer together. The chapter ends with the plan of the book.

Reclaiming professionalism

Richardson (1989) draws our attention to the bureaucratisation of social services departments. This relates not only to their size (the 'Seebohm factories' as they have been called), but also to the ways in which they have 'established policies and structures which induce conformity and reduce professional autonomy' (Richardson, 1989: 123). Whilst some professional groups 'retain considerable degrees of autonomy, the ability to define and determine clients' needs and treatments and a role in policy determination' (Cousins, 1987: 91), others, the semi-professions, are 'more vulnerable to the extension of managerial controls or subordination by the established professions' (Cousins, 1987: 91).

Professions, as well as bureaucratic management, are engaged in processes of control and conformity. The welfare professions have been criticised for their concern with status, privilege, gatekeeping, and their development of expert models of practice that serve to enhance the power of the professional over the consumer (Cousins, 1987; Illich et al, 1977). Research evidence has shown that professional assessments of need arise from a mix of professional worker values and routine practices of the organisation. And routine practices have been shown to reflect patterns of power and dominant values in organisations (Foucault, 1980). Assessment is seldom undertaken through rigorous and theoretical analysis (Smith and Harris, 1972). As Sinfield warned us in 1969, at the beginning of the post-Seebohm area:

> The firm establishment of a profession may lead to the strengthening of the professional in defence of his client, to higher quality

in work and a greater assumption of responsibilities. But equally professionalisation may bring dangers, coming between the worker and his client or the community at large. Unification may serve a multitude of purposes.... It may strengthen the professional against the bureaucrat, but also against the public, and may help to legitimise demands for further privileges, rights and benefits to be awarded in deference to assured professional status. (Sinfield, 1969: 23–4)

Welfare professionalism needs to be reclaimed from managerialism and from the 'bourgeois improvers' (Smith, 1988: 143). To be emancipatory it needs to be autonomous of both and concerned with the practice of its craft. In his foreword to *Child Care Research, Policy and Practice*, Utting reminds us that:

Being professional imposes, among other requirements, the responsibility of keeping up to date with professional developments, extending knowledge and improving skills in one's chosen craft. Conscientious application to the lessons of relevant research is an essential part of this process. (Utting, 1989: vii)

If the purpose of the craft of the welfare professional is to strive towards human well-being, justice and equality, then intellectual work and research is fundamental to reveal the structures and mechanisms that generate and maintain inequality:

Intellectual work is related to power in numerous ways, among them these: with ideas one can uphold or justify power, attempting to transform it into legitimate authority; with ideas one can also debunk authority, attempting to reduce it to mere power, to discredit it as arbitrary or as unjust. With ideas one can conceal or expose the holders of power. And with ideas of more hypnotic though frivolous shape, one can divert attention from problems of power and authority and social reality in general. (Mills, 1963: 612)

Further, practitioners must be concerned with developing knowledge in ways which enable users of social services, as well as providers, to become 'knowers'. As recipients of social work services, their understandings of their experiences of social inequality need to be acknowledged as legitimate. Sinfield proposes the social worker as 'social investigator' to report back on the faults in the organisation of our society and the distribution of its goods and services (Sinfield, 1969).

The research-minded practitioner

Our experience and our examples are based in social work. However, we envisage that, in the broad approach we take to social work, this book may be useful to other professionals: health visitors, teachers, youth workers, community workers, adult education and play workers. Being research-minded is relevant to other professional areas. Smith, for example, in his writing about youth workers, argues that

> it is sustained reflection and dialogue over time which provides the most potential, especially where this is based upon the exploration of actual and continuing practice and the traditions which it expresses. It is essential that things are not taken at their face value and that the hidden structures are sought; the underlying reasons for intervention require careful thought. (Smith, 1988, 142–3)

Research-minded practice is concerned with the analytical assessment of social need and resources, and the development, implementation and evaluation of strategies to meet that need. It is not constrained by organisational and professional boundaries. Hence the research-minded practitioner does not necessarily deliver the service or apply the therapeutic technique that is expected in the routine processes of the organisation and the profession: service delivery for elderly people, group work for young offenders, family therapy in situations of child abuse. The taken-for-granted becomes subject to critical scrutiny. An examination of research methodology and exploration of research methods is fundamental to such practice. For such a practitioner,

> Research is an intellectual journey in which the researchers must constantly engage with their purposes, subject, theories, methods and data. The constant interaction between reading, thinking, perusing materials and data, analysing etc is the essence of research activity. (Hardiker, 1989: 6)

Thus, research-minded practitioners:

- will be constantly defining and making explicit their objectives and hypotheses;
- will treat their explanations of the social world as hypotheses – that is, as tentative and open to be tested against evidence;

- will be aware of their expertise and knowledge and that of others;
- will bring to the fore theories that help make sense of social need, resources and assist in decision making with regard to strategies;
- will be thoughtful, reflecting on data and theory and contributing to their development and refinement;
- will scrutinise and be analytical of available data and information;
- will be mindful of the pervasiveness of ideology and values in the way we see and understand the world.

The social work experience of research

For many practitioners, research conjures up statistics, experiments, questionnaires. For example, a commonly held view in social work is that 'science deals splendidly with all that can be weighed, measured or counted, but this involves excluding from the universe of discourse the intangible, the imponderable, all that cannot be reduced to statistics' (Irvine, 1969: 4). Similarly, Goldberg, a prolific social work researcher with a background in epidemiology, wrote:

Putting people into categories and quantifying phenomena, which in the last analysis are subjective experiences, cuts right across the social worker's belief in the uniqueness of individual experiences and the need to individualise problems in order to help people in their difficulties. (Goldberg, 1972: 139)

In the same vein, Shaw (1975) suggests that the objectivity of science seems inferior to the warmth and spontaneity of social worker/client relationships. And more recently, in 1985, Sainsbury, commenting that 'the relationship between research and practice is ambiguous', compares social work practice with that of research describing the former as taking place 'in situations of conflicting values, ambivalent motivations and ambiguous social demands [providing for the researcher] an unwieldy number of variables, many of which may not even be recognised, let alone controlled' (Sainsbury 1985: 5).

At best, practitioners experience research as irrelevant; at worst, as the process of being ripped off. In other words, practitioners and their practice may be used for research purposes which may not necessarily enhance practice.

To be able to encompass research activity as part of the repertoire of the practitioner, it is important critically to reflect on these notions of research. This requires an understanding of issues of epistemology and methodology. In this chapter these are introduced to enable the reader to stand back from what he or she may perhaps have always thought of, and rejected, as research. They are pursued in more detail in the following chapter. Epistemology is the study of theories of knowledge. What is knowledge? What can we know about the social world? Who can become knowledgeable? What do we choose to know? How do we get to know? These are important epistemological and methodological questions. Methodology is the study of theories of methods. Methods are the techniques of doing research: asking questions, observing people and groups, analysing case records, sifting through historical documents and local newspapers.

In the Western world, research is largely undertaken in the positivist tradition. The market research social survey is the most common form of research activity. Positivism is an epistemology, a collection of theories of knowledge. There are many versions of positivism. Fundamentally, positivist theories treat the social sciences like the natural and physical sciences. We can become knowledgeable about the social world as we do about the natural and physical one. Social data are facts that can be gathered, through value free observation and listening. What is more, they can be gathered in such a way that our fingerprints do not leave any trace on them. In other words, they remain uncontaminated by the gathering process. Thus positivist researchers believe that their understandings and experiences of the world do not affect what they observe and hear. They would take issue with the contention of C. Wright Mills (1963) that intellectual work is related to power and legitimacy.

Positivists not only see their work as uncontaminated: they see themselves as pure and safe in their objectivity, an elite who have managed to transcend the constraints of subjectivity. Data collection methods are structured to eliminate or control for the influence of intervening variables, such as the researcher. Data, as social facts, may be analysed quantitatively. They can be measured, added up, related to each other causally and controlled in experiments. Statistical techniques are developed to analyse the probability of findings being true.

In this introductory chapter, we contrast positivist styles with interpretive and critical styles of research. Interpretive epistemologies reject the possibility of objective social facts. Rather, social phenomena are given meanings by those who define and make them explicit. Thus different people will have different subjective understandings of social phenomena. In its extreme, such an approach hardly allows for the possibility of research. Each person has their own subjective understanding and experience of the social world and all we can hope for is knowledge of our own subjectivity through contemplation. Interpretive methodologists believe, however, that it is possible to research subjectivities.

Critical theorists disagree with both positivists and interpretists. They do not believe in the existence of social facts. Neither do they take the other extreme of subjectivity. Critical theorists argue that there are social patterns, structures which shape our subjective understandings of the world. We can understand the meanings of different people's subjectivities by relating them to social structures such as class, race and gender. Thus critical theorists theorise subjectivities.

As the social survey is the hallmark of positivist social research, so ethnography is for interpretists and critical theorists. Ethnography is concerned with the study of everyday life in natural settings. Participant observation, where the researcher participates in the activity, is a common method of collecting data for ethnographic studies.

Chapter 2 explains in more detail these and other competing epistemologies. Already though, it should have occurred to the reader that there is a better philosophical and methodological fit between the more interpretive and critical epistemologies and social work theories and methods than between social work and positivism. The relationship between social work and research may be enhanced by conceptualising and practising research within an epistemology other than positivism.

In saying this, we do not reject positivist styles of research. They can be of value to social welfare. We only need to reflect on the significance of studies of poverty and health inequality to appreciate that positivist research can be extremely important in promoting justice and social welfare (Townsend and Davidson, 1982; Townsend, Phillimore and Beattie, 1988). The point we make is that positivist styles of research do not fit easily with styles of practice. Other styles may open up possibilities and opportunities for practitioners to incorporate research into their routine work.

We continue by exploring further why it is that social work has clung to positivist notions of research when the social sciences have been rapidly rejecting them – in theory anyway. We then explore the research tradition in social work and developments that have taken place concerned, intentionally or not, with enhancing research in social work. Amongst these developments are those within humanistic enquiry and feminist research. Such approaches to research open up exciting possibilities for the practitioner who is research-minded.

Social work's research tradition

In theoretical debates within the social sciences today positivism is regarded sceptically. An understanding of the relationship between our place in society and how we see the social world, recognising society as stratified by gender, race, class and age, leads to a questioning of the notion of value-free observation. In seeking to understand social workers' antipathy towards research, what is interesting is that, although the dominant theoretical paradigm in the social sciences is no longer positivist, the predominant ways in which research is carried out continue to be in this tradition. Platt found this to be the case in her analysis of research published in the main sociological journals. She accounts for this thus: first, those who do research and get research published are senior in their professional and academic careers and operate within former dominant paradigms; second, the methods of researchers are more influenced by the bodies which fund and sponsor research than by their own theoretical ideas; third, positivist styles of research, or quantitative research, will be what is expected of policy research and what is respected by policy makers and managers (Platt, 1981).

Social work's disengagement from research is, we suggest, a disengagement from positivism. We have already shown how researchers in social work contrast research with social work. They suggest that research is often quantitative, objective and concerned with social categories. They contrast this with social work which is uncertain, complex, spontaneous and concerned with individual difference. In this they perceive research within the positivist paradigm. It may indeed be the case that much of social work research is positivist, for the reasons suggested by Platt (1981), and that social work research, based both in social administration and medical epidemiology, has been constrained by the positivist models of these disciplines.

It has been suggested that the gap between social work and research is one of immaturity, that social work still has to come of age as a profession; that this ageing process will encompass a research base of some strength (Hanvey, 1990). However, reflecting on the history of social work reveals a time past when social work and social research were very much interrelated. In fact, Clement Attlee, then a social work lecturer at the London School of Economics, described

> social investigation [as] a particular form of social work . . . It is not possible for the ordinary rank and file of social workers to hope to rival skilled investigators, but each one can take his part by cultivating habits of careful observation and analysis of the pieces of social machinery that come under his notice. (Attlee, 1920: 230, quoted in Sinfield, 1969: 53)

At the beginning of this century, the relationship between social administration and social work, and thus between social work and policy research, was strong. This policy research was fundamentally positivist. Finch traces policy research to its roots in the nineteenth-century statistical societies, the poverty studies of Booth and Rowntree and the work of the Webbs. This research, primarily the poverty surveys published in 'blue books', to become known as 'blue book sociology', was grounded in

> the impartial collection of facts; an unproblematic conception of 'facts', based on a positivist epistemology; a belief in the direct utility of such facts in shaping measures of social reform which can be implemented by governments; and a strong preference for statistical methods and the social survey as the most suitable technique for fact-collecting. (Finch, 1986: 37)

What is less often recalled is that there were significant qualitative, social philosophical and socially committed elements to this research activity. Booth gathered qualitative as well as quantitative data, taking lodgings in the poor areas of his studies and undertaking covert participant observation. He also engaged School Board Visitors in his research activity. It was they, the educational welfare officers of the turn of the century, who were the researchers for Booth's work, who provided the research data for the studies of the extent and causes of poverty. Such was the involvement of 'social workers' in research. Beatrice Webb worked as one of

Booth's interviewers and was herself critical of the static picture presented by the positivist social survey. Octavia Hill and Helen Bosanquet both insisted on getting to know the poor to understand them. What they did not do, however, was to conceptualise their work as research. They did not name their work as ethnographic, as indeed, with hindsight, it was. The work that was recognised as research was that which adopted a positivist epistemology and it was this approach to research that was to remain predominant in social administration research. The work of Octavia Hill and Helen Bosanquet was to become equated with social work. It is interesting to reflect on the fit between the work of women and qualitative approaches to understanding and social work; and the fit between men, quantitative measures and social research.

The Webbs and the Bosanquets combined intellectual work, research, social action and social work. This combination of theory, practice and social intervention was the strength of the Department of Social Administration at the London School of Economics which was formed in 1912 out of the School of Sociology of the Charity Organisation Society (COS) and the Ratan Tata poverty research unit (Harris, 1989: 27–63). Social work and social policy practice were one, informed through rigorous theoretical analysis and empirical work. This is not to say that there were not theoretical and ideological tensions between them: tensions between theory and practice, between empirical work and value commitments, between collectivism and individualism. Recent evidence has come to light to suggest, however, that these were tensions of no greater order than the bread and butter of debate in any academic community (Harris,1989).

Social work and social policy were in some ways to part company and develop separately. To some extent this was to the detriment of both: social policy developed as atheoretical empiricism – fact gathering without the theoretical frameworks to make sense of, and judge between, facts (Mishra, 1989). Social work narrowed to 'its current more isolated and residual position' (Bulmer, Lewis and Piachaud, 1989: 11; Pinker, 1989).

There is no necessary link, of course, between, on the one hand, the move away from social and political theory and commitment to social change, and on the other, a rejection of research. As social work became medicalised and therapeutic, so it could have taken on epidemiological and experimental approaches to the development of its knowledge base. And indeed there have been significant attempts in this direction. What we have attempted to demonstrate in this section is that there was once a vibrant relationship between social work and social research. And we unashamedly argue for a revival of such an approach to social work research, this time geared to more explicitly emancipatory ends: an approach that has been described as one of 'passionate scholarship' (du Bois, 1983).

Developments in research for social change

There have been a number of significant developments in research that might have enhanced the relationship between social work and social research. The exploration of these introduces us to debates in research methodology and policy research which help inform our development of a methodology for the research-minded practitioner.

The National Community Development Project (CDP) was launched in 1969 as a government experiment to address pockets of deprivation in twelve local authority areas. They were experiments too in combining social action with social research, in action–research. Each of the twelve projects had a research team provided by a neighbouring academic institution. The research methodology was that of action–research, drawing from the experience of the Educational Priority Areas (Halsey, 1972), the American War on Poverty (Marris and Rein, 1967) and, perhaps less well known but significant for social work, the Family Advice Services project (Leissner, Herdman and Davies, 1971).

The Home Office model of action-research was informed by positivism:

> whereby expert researchers would identify the social problems of
> . an area (using 'objective' techniques of measurement such as
> social surveys and official statistics, in the best positivist tradi-
> tion), then community workers would move in to implement
> strategies for ameliorative action based on this research; the
> research team would then have the task of expertly and objec-
> tively monitoring different strategies for intervention. (Chapman
> and Green, 1990: 3)

At the time, stories from the CDPs on the relationship between the action workers and the research workers were rife. There were cases where the research team was reputed to have been thrown out of the project by the action team for its insistence on conducting positivist-style neighbourhood social surveys when the action team expected research more dynamically linked with the immediacy of action. At the other extreme were the projects in which action and research workers joined together in action–research, engaging in community development to analyse and understand how some communities come to be deprived. What is particularly interesting for us is that they

> rejected the Home Office's distinction between action and research.... It was partly a methodological argument about the nature of research as a means of obtaining knowledge about social and economic reality. Some members of the Tyneside CDPs, for example, claimed to base their version of 'action-research' on Habermas's critical theory, which involved a denial of the objective–subjective dichotomy and its replacement by a view of the researcher as actively engaging with the social reality that he/she is trying at the same time to interpret and to change. (Chapman and Green, 1990: 4)

Thus the CDPs contained a significant element that brought research and practice together. Whereas Habermas argues for the researcher to be engaged with action (Habermas, 1974), we argue in this book for the practitioner to be engaged with research. *The development of research in social work organisations* followed the publication of the Seebohm report. Some of the newly formed social services departments established research units 'to furnish management with data needed for policy making' (CCETSW/PSSC, 1980: 5). The model of research and planning advocated by the DHSS to guide these new research workers was again one of positivism. These early researchers, at a significant time when they were marking out the territory for in-house research, became embroiled in the construction of the Ten Year Plans (Booth, 1988) and the undertaking of social surveys to implement Section I of the Chronically Sick and Disabled Persons Act (Jaehnig, 1973). Similarly, the research sections of Probation Services became concerned mainly with the production of official data for the Home Office and the testing out of performance review techniques.

The impact of these in-house research units on the work of practitioners, with a few exceptions (see, for example, Addison and Rosen, 1985), was marginal. Voluntary agencies have also developed in-house research units. Some have made significant efforts to ensure that research staff relate, not only to managers to assist them with planning and the effective allocation of scarce resources, but also to practitioners to help them build evaluation into their service delivery and practice. Policy developments within community care, the National Health Service and Community Care Act 1990, and the 1989 Children Act bring with them increasing emphasis on inspection and quality assurance. This relates to both statutory services and private, independent and voluntary organisations with whom contracts or working agreements are made for the delivery of services. We would argue that it is important that practitioners are involved in such developments and that inspection and quality control are linked with practitioner evaluation (Everitt et al, 1991). In our model research for quality must not be equated with research for management for rational decision making.

The teaching of research to social workers has taken place within qualifying and post qualifying social work courses and through the provision of short courses. This has sometimes been with the intention of enabling those qualifying in social work to understand research, sometimes to conduct research as part of their practice, and sometimes, particularly within four year degree programmes, to appreciate the problematical nature of knowledge (Everitt 1982). The validating body, the Central Council for Education and Training in Social Work (CCETSW), although in the past somewhat ambivalent about whether research is appropriate for the qualifying practitioner, has more recently been much more encouraging of educationalists wanting to adopt such an approach:

> Qualifying social workers need a rigorous approach to the acquisition of knowledge. They must become confident in identifying, locating and using relevant source material – factual, general, specialist and research. They must be able to conceptualise, to reflect, to analyse competing theories, ideologies, and models of practice which will inform their work. (CCETSW, 1989: 14).

A research route for the Advanced Award is recommended. Whitaker and Archer (1989) have made a valuable contribution in demystifying research for social work practitioners to enable them to undertake pieces of research.

Research dissemination exercises have been significant particularly in the child care field. The House of Commons, Social Services Committee, in its report on the Children in Care investigation, drew attention to the inconsistency of research in child care and the lack of influence of research findings on the practice of social workers

(House of Commons 1984; Kahan 1989). Through the Social Service Inspectorate, the DHSS has undertaken dissemination exercises, publishing synopses of child care research (DHSS, 1985) and convening regional seminars for practitioners, managers, policy makers and educationalists. *Child Care Research, Policy and Practice* is yet another contribution to 'the dissemination process and in attempting to make research "user friendly" the style and language used are directed to non-academic readers primarily, it being well established that the language and presentation of academic research reports do not encourage wide readership' (Kahan, 1989: 2).

Given the concerted attempts that have been made to publicise, understand and consider the implications of findings from child care research, it is interesting to reflect on the extent to which research has influenced legislation with the passing of the 1989 Children Act (Harwin, 1990).

The participative research movement recognises the relationship between research, knowledge and power. The Association of Researchers in Voluntary Action (ARVAC) and the Participatory Research Exchange have provided a valuable educative and supportive service and helped disseminate participatory research ideas. In participatory research, the subjects of research are involved in the research process. In Chapter 4, we take this model as a basis for developing the notion of the research-minded practitioner. In participatory research, the essential relationship between research process and the research task is addressed through its primary method, dialogue. Data are created through discussion amongst all participants in the process of service delivery: users, practitioners, managers and workers from other agencies. The intention of participatory research is to democratise the research process, to achieve greater equality between the researcher and the researched (Croft and Beresford, 1984). This model of research provides opportunities for bringing the practice of the crafts of social welfare and social research closer together.

The development of feminist research has many links with participatory research, particularly in its conceptualising, both theoretically and politically, a different relationship between objectivity and subjectivity in research. Feminist researchers are concerned to develop research processes that neither neglect women nor objectify them (Stanley and Wise, 1983). So, within feminism, as in the critical approach and in participatory research, the subjects of the research, that is those from whom data are sought, become fully

2

Epistemology and Theory in Social Work

Research is a publicly accountable activity. As such it contrasts with 'intuition', with taken-for-granted assumptions that remain private and implicit, and with 'common sense'. Practitioners who are research-minded seriously appraise their understandings of the world. They consider how these are shaped through personal experience in specific historical, social and economic contexts. They reflect on the way these understandings relate to their practice. This requires that practitioners are clear and open about the theories they bring into play.

Theory is important in understanding the complexities of need and social problems and in deciding how to address these effectively. Practitioners must pay attention to theory in order to explain to themselves, to managers, to other workers and to users how they have come to particular understandings and decisions about practice. They need to do this in order 'to make informed choices, to keep up to date with advances and to discard redundant theories' (Hardiker and Barker, 1991: 87). If they do not, practitioners are in danger of accepting uncritically common sense and organisational routine ways of approaching their work.

To summarise, then, practitioners need to pay attention to:

- theories that inform their assessments and analyses of need and social problems;
- theories that influence their decisions about services and interventions, and their effectiveness;
- theories that underpin their very approaches to becoming, and their claims to be, knowledgeable – or, in other words, to epistemology (theories of knowledge).

involved in the research process. Attention is paid to t
understandings and experiences of both the researc
researched in a process of sharing and exploring m
ther. Feminists have theorised the relationship between
and the political, private and public, between su
objective. Through theory and empirical work, the f
mies between these have been demonstrated. New wa
at the world have emerged through recognising that th
one, for example the personal, can only be underst
reference to the other, that is the political. Feminis
make use of a range of methods producing both qu
quantitative data (another false dichotomy) to facilit
dialogue. Fundamental to feminist research is its purp
both its process and its task, to address gender inequa
research methodology is compatible with the craft of s
practice that has as its purpose human well-being
equality.

Plan of the book

We attempt to develop a social work methodology inf
work of researchers, by learning from their triump
failures. The book is in two parts. In this chapter,
following, we work towards the development of a met
the practitioner who is research-minded. Chapter 2
epistemology in social work and Chapter 3 address
chapters 4 to 8, we explore the process of practice
research-mindedness. Chapter 4 is concerned with la
model for such a practice. Pursuing this model, in C
suggest ways in which the research-minded practition
issues. Chapter 6 explores ways in which the rese
practitioner engages with subjects to generate und
Chapter 7 is concerned with analysis, while Chapte
the notion of the practitioner–evaluator. A short c
presented in the last chapter.

In this chapter we attempt to demonstrate how crucial epistemological theory is in social work. Different ways of knowing and understanding the world make different assumptions about the individual and society, and about their interrelationships. Unless these assumptions are teased out, they may be adopted unknowingly and uncritically by practitioners. And yet these assumptions have implications for practice.

If the fundamental purpose of social welfare is the pursuit of justice and equality, then practitioners have a professional responsibility to be alert to the ways in which power operates through ways of knowing. To be in a position to understand and name the needs and problems that others experience is to be powerful. To be in a position where others accord you the right to know and give credibility to your understandings, is also powerful. And it is especially powerful to be able to secure, through legal requirement or voluntarily, the engagement of others in a range of mechanisms and approaches, treatments and care plans, on the basis of these understandings. As Worrall points out in relation to theorising the experiences of women who offend against the law:

> The relationship between knowledge and power is crucial to any attempt to theorize women's experiences. The desire to know is a desire for power but knowledge of itself does not give power. On the contrary, it is those who have power who are authorised 'to know' and whose 'knowledge' is afforded privilege (Worrall, 1990: 7).

The issue of legitimacy helps us further to understand what kinds of knowledge, and whose, effectively define situations. People habitually use many different ways of knowing, but prioritise their sources differently. For many people, what others tell them, particularly if those others are in positions of power, is considered more important than what they know themselves. For other people, their own feelings are taken far more seriously than any other kind of evidence. In general, the more socially unacceptable the knowledge, the greater the burden of proof that will be required of the messenger. Social work is an area in which many unwanted truths have to be addressed. One of the main challenges for the practitioner who is research-minded is to develop an epistemological understanding of the processes by which unwanted truths remain hidden from those who cannot or do not wish to face their implications. This can only proceed from a clear consideration of the practitioner's own value base and the broader social context.

Research-minded practitioners would see it as fundamental to tease out ways in which they understand and define the world of others: to reveal the social sources and social consequences of their knowledge for analysis and debate. Research-minded practitioners would accord others with whom they work the right to know, and would accord service users the right to know about their own lives. This was the purpose of Worrall's study of women who offend against the law (Worrall, 1990), and is introduced by Cain and Smart thus:

> [Worrall] looks at what passes for knowledge about such women. This knowledge she identifies as part of the regulation of these women, it is also a part of their silencing. Women who offend are silenced, they become muted and unable to provide their own accounts of their subjectivity. The experts always already know these women and, through this knowledge, seek to manage them. (Cain and Smart, in Worrall, 1990: viii)

Professional ways of knowing in our society have served to objectify and control others. Professionals are regarded as knowledgeable: others are objects of this knowledge. In this chapter we will explore ways in which people do understand their own lives, ways in which subjectivities are constructed.

Key ideas and concepts in theorising ways of knowing

In the first chapter we introduced theories of knowledge. Inter-pretive methodologies take account of subjectivities, of the influence of the values, beliefs and perspectives of the 'knower' in what is claimed to be known. Critical methodologies place subjectivities in their social context, recognising the social processes and social structures through which people come to understand the world in a particular way. Positivist methodologies assume that 'reality' exists independently of the 'knower', the person constructing it, independent of the subject. And positivists assume that conclusions about 'reality' may be objectively drawn without reference either to meaning assigned to it by the 'knower' or to the context in which it has been constructed. Further, positivists seek data about, and manipulate, variables in such a way that causal relationships between them may be made. Explanations are sought about what causes certain phenomena. The next step is to be able to argue that, if one variable exists, or a particular cluster of variables exist, then certain things will follow. In other words, predictions may be made. On the basis of these predictions, interventions may be chosen to effect particular changes and outcomes. This is, of course, of particular relevance to the practitioner – knowing the world in order effectively to intervene in it.

In place of positivism, we have argued that ways in which social work practitioners understand the world probably fit better with theories of knowledge that take account of subjectivities and of the social processes through which they are constructed. This has been well expressed by the psychologist and counsellor, Carl Rogers (1967), in considering the development of his own theory and practice. He points out the conflict between positivism and his perspective in the following way:

> I can recognise the origin of the conflicts. It was between the logical positivism in which I was educated, for which I had a deep respect, and the subjectively oriented existential thinking which was taking root in me because it seemed to fit so well with my therapeutic experience. (Rogers, 1967: 199)

It is our contention that: (1) epistemologies that take account of the processes and structures through which subjective understandings of the world are formed; and (2) methodologies that create and validate data through participatory processes are compatible with social welfare practice. These contrast with epistemologies and methodologies from which practitioners have become alienated: those which engage in processes of research that, in striving for objectivity, seek distance between the researcher and the researched and attempt to control for social variables, including the researcher, lest they contaminate the data collected.

One thing needs to be clarified though. Positivism relates to an epistemological position. The term is also used at times to describe quantitative research – or, to be more precise, research that produces data that are analysed quantitatively and statistically. Thus positivism and quantitative research are sometimes equated with each other. Whilst social workers may be uncomfortable with an epistemology that seeks to control variables in the elusive quest for objectivity, they may, at the same time, find quantitative data and statistical analysis useful. Also certain methods believed to be

intrinsically positivist may provide valuable qualitative data. For
example, data generated through focused interviews in social
surveys may provide rich material from which qualitative categories can be derived (Hardiker and Barker, 1986); and research that
takes account of subjective understandings, and the social processes
and contexts through which data are constructed, may well produce
data that can be quantified.

Researchers who criticise positivism argue that reality cannot be
defined or understood independently of the 'knower', the person
studying or constructing it: that 'reality' is socially constructed.
Understandings, rather than explanations, of the world are sought.
Extreme interpretists believe that reality can only be individually
known. The possibilities of a science of society are then limited to
individual reflection. The possibilities for free will and autonomous
creative thought are great. Critical theorists, though, both Marxists
and feminists, would argue that individual interpretations of the
world, subjective interpretations, can be understood by reference to
the social contexts in which they have been formed. Thus, class,
gender and race, for example, structure the ways in which we
experience and make sense of the world. Autonomous creative
thought is limited by social structures and processes.

The debates are about the possibility of an objective reality, one
that exists independently of the 'knower' and the interpreter, or one
that can be understood through the analysis of subjectivities. These
debates have been extended by the argument that it is language that
creates phenomena through the process of naming and that it is
language that defines our thoughts and ideas: language is said to
construct 'reality' rather than to 'reflect' it (Rojek, Peacock and
Collins, 1988: 144). The social processes and structures that social
constructionists regard as significant in forming our ideas and
perceptions are themselves structured through discourses, through
sets of languages, concepts and codes. These discourses therefore
need to be subject to the same processes of deconstruction as do
positivist realities.

We illustrate this with the example of 'race'. In being research-
minded in our practice, it would be important to take account of
'race'. If we do not, then we will find ourselves colluding with
institutional racism: that is, discriminating against people who are
black by only addressing the needs and resources of the dominant
majority white community; allowing discriminatory systems in
education, housing, criminal justice and so on to take their
course; uncritically adopting stereotypical views about the lives

and experiences of people who are black. For critical theorists, it would be important to take account of 'race' in its structuring of our experiences, and ideas and perceptions, of the world. To grow up black in Western society is significantly different from being white. Racism ensures that black children have different educational experiences, black young people experience the process of getting a job differently, and they experience the criminal justice system differently. Black feminists have made an extremely significant contribution to feminist theory and research by clearly showing that it is not only gender but 'race' as well that must be taken into account in revealing and understanding the place of women in our society.

But what is 'race'? It is 'merely' a construct in our society used to categorise people, to make differences between people, to discriminate between people on account of these differences, and to exercise control over people. In using the word 'merely', we are not suggesting that 'race' is insignificant. Far from it. 'Race' is so pervasive as a construct, so effective in its naming and defining of people, that people's experiences are indeed structured through its application. Its very pervasiveness in our experiences, in our language, influences and is influenced by the development of a taken-for-granted common sense: one in which it is assumed, unless challenged, that 'race' is a real, natural phenomenon, that people are divided into 'races' naturally. Processes of knowledge making have contributed to this common sense about 'race': 'the notion of race has been the subject of much pseudo-scientific thinking, which has influenced public consciousness' (Giddens, 1989: 246). Our word 'merely' is there to signify that 'race' is not real. There are as many genetic differences between people who share certain physical attributes as between groups divided by 'race'.

These facts lead many biologists, 'anthropologists and sociologists to believe that the concept of race should be dropped altogether' (Giddens, 1989: 246). People are different in their physical appearances: that some of these differences are chosen to be significant and used to divide people is to do with power, not to do with biology. There is an answer to 'it's only natural': and that is, 'its to do with power and discrimination'. 'Race' is not real and natural: it is a discourse of values, assumptions, language, theories and practices that comes to be experienced as real. If discourses, such as 'race', are to do with power, they are also however to do with resistance. The concept of 'race' is deployed to discriminate against people who are black. It is also deployed by black people to resist and challenge this power. Black movements, and black projects in social welfare, are important in the work they do to challenge 'race'. (For further discussion of the deployment of the concept of 'race' by black groups, see Fuss, 1989: 73–96.)

This example has illustrated that being research-minded in practice means thinking epistemologically about what we have come to know and how we have come to understand the world. If we do not think critically in these ways, then we are in danger of taking for granted the commonsense way of seeing things. Common sense constitutes predominant views in society. And in an unequal society divided by race, class, gender, sexuality, age and able-bodiedness, these views will in themselves be imbued with discriminatory notions. Common sense views need to be analysed and deconstructed. This is a responsibility of a practitioner who is research-minded.

Theoretical perspectives in social work

In social work there have been a number of important attempts to develop frameworks to serve as guides for practitioners in their exploration of theory and its relevance and validity for practice (Hardiker and Barker, 1981; Bailey and Lee, 1982; Howe, 1987; Roberts, 1990; Payne 1991). These studies have classified theories in a number of ways. They have been concerned with the elaboration of theories developed directly to inform practice, prescribing different approaches for social workers to adopt, such as task-centred casework theories, behavioural social work theories and systemic theories. Analyses of theories have also been concerned with teasing out more fundamental theoretical approaches assumed within them. These fundamental theories may adopt contrasting views of the individual and society and their interrelationship. They also may understand the process of 'getting to know' differently. Leonard (1975) distinguishes between those within a physical science paradigm (positivism) and those within a human sciences paradigm (interpretist and critical theories) (see also Howe, 1987). These analyses of social work theories have demonstrated that:

● there is not one way of understanding the world and of deciding upon courses of action;
● different theoretical perspectives have different implications for practice, thus making it necessary for practitioners to be open

with themselves and with others about which ones they are
employing;
● theories are based upon different assumptions concerning how
we know about the social world;
● theories make different assumptions about the nature of the
individual and society;
● perhaps most importantly of all, theories make different
assumptions about the nature of change in society and how
this may occur and be promoted.

In this chapter on epistemology and theory we examine psychoanalytic, Marxist and feminist theoretical approaches as fundamental underpinning theories. We choose these because:

● they adopt different perspectives on the ways in which subjectivities are shaped;
● they are all concerned with developing understandings of the
construction of individual consciousness in order to engage in
emancipatory practice;
● they all have influenced social work theory and practice.

In line with the purpose of this book, our particular interest in
exploring these theoretical approaches is to consider the validity of
their claims to know and to consider ways in which they help us
judge what others profess to know. For the practitioner who is
research-minded, these issues about knowledge, and judging the
truth of that knowledge, are of key importance.

We have suggested that positivism, as a way of knowing about
the world, is not the most appropriate epistemology for social work.
If we reject positivism as a theory of knowledge and a methodology
for getting to know, then it behoves us to be clear about the claims
to knowledge that we do make. What legitimacy do we have for
having, and being accorded, professional authority? What legitimacy do we have for intervening? If we profess to engage in practice
that is emancipatory, then it is particularly important that we
address these questions.

What distinguishes theoretical knowledge from ideology and
common sense? How do we judge the validity of different claims
to knowledge? What claims to knowledge are made within psychoanalysis, Marxism and feminism? These are the questions we will
begin to tackle in this chapter. And we will return to them in
Chapter 7 when we consider how research-minded practitioners

might understand and analyse data generated through their practice.

We will not come up with final answers. These are questions which have long taunted philosophers, epistemologists and scientists. It is important, nevertheless, that research-minded practitioners turn their attention to the validity and partiality of their claims to know – and the claims to know that others profess (users, managers, workers in other agencies). Can I claim that the way I understand the world, what I see as happening, is somehow right? What accord do I give to other people's understandings? Do I only go along with them if their views fit mine? Or do I take a relativist approach – everybody understands the world differently and that's fine? How do I then make judgements between different views? Before we can answer these questions we need to tease out and understand how we, and others, approach the world. What theoretical perspectives do we adopt to understand the ways in which we, and others, come to hold particular views?

Psychodynamic perspectives

There are many schools of psychodynamic thought that stem from Freud's theories of psychoanalysis. Fundamental to them all is the assumption of the existence of unconscious mental processes which can be studied through the exploration of the subjective. The unconscious for Freud was biological and instinctual. Post-Freudians have placed more stress on other factors which influence the unconscious: social and cultural factors and factors associated with interpersonal relations. Freud himself claimed validity for his theory and research by recourse to his scientific method. He was a positivist, a natural scientist who sought evidence of causal relationships between the unconscious and behaviour, and between sexuality in childhood and the development of personality. Freud's clinical method of research, his way of collecting data, was through the analysis of dreams, fantasies, word-associations, slips of the tongue and thoughts expressed while under hypnosis. He objectified the person, 'the patient', in positivist mode, by interpreting these data within his own theoretical frameworks.

Freud's scientific claim to validity and his objectifying of the 'patient' has been subject to considerable debate amongst psychoanalysts. They have pursued the same debate that has taken place between positivists and interpretists throughout the social sciences:

in recent years, some analysts . . . have held that psychoanalysis is not an *eklartung* psychology (concerned with explanation) but a *verstehende* psychology (concerned with understanding). It is best regarded, they would hold, as a semantic rather than a causal theory, concerned essentially with meaning and with the intuitive understanding of the individual's perceptions and values and the intensely subjective and personal world in which he moves, which is shaped in part by his biographical experiences. The task of the analyst is to enter this subjective world . . . (Yelloly, 1980: 159, emphasis in original)

Notwithstanding this debate, theories of the unconscious provided explanations for seemingly random and irrational behaviour that rationalist psychologists had found difficult to explain. Or, in other words, psychoanalytic theory, and the theoretical construct the unconscious, seemed to work and to provide better understandings than those that had come before.

The important ways in which psychoanalytic theories have contributed to the understandings and interventions of social workers have been well documented (Yelloly, 1980; Pearson, Treseder and Yelloly, 1988; Brearley, 1991). These writers suggest that psychoanalytic theory has had considerable influence upon the way social workers think, mainly through its being so pervasive in Western discourse. As it has become part of Western culture, so it has also become part of social work. However, the practice of psychoanalysis has had less impact on what social workers do:

it is essential to draw a clear distinction between the contribution of psychoanalysis to the understanding of human behaviour and emotional life, and its contribution to the methodology of social work. Its impact on the former has in my view been by far the greatest; the treatment techniques of psychoanalysis lie well outside what social work regards as its territorial waters. (Yelloly, 1980: 166)

For social work, psychoanalysis has been useful in its focusing on the potential influence of past and forgotten events and of experiences of childhood on current behaviour and emotions (Yelloly, 1980: 26). It is concerned with the relationships between self and significant other people – past and present experience – inner and outer reality (Brearley, 1991: 49–50). It has also been used by Menzies (1988) to enhance understandings of the dynamics of organisations. We can tease out psychoanalytically influenced thinking when we come across the social worker who seeks explanations for a person's behaviour and feelings in their history and experiences, particularly in early childhood, and in the social worker who regards intra-psychic processes, or, in other words, what goes on inside a person's mind, as more important than any extra-psychic circumstances, the social context.

Psychoanalytic perspectives would alert the research-minded practitioner to factors in their own childhood and past, and possibly forgotten, experiences, that may influence their understanding of the world. So too, these perspectives would raise similar questions for the way users understand their experiences and interpret what is happening in their lives. An understanding of the unconscious would encourage the research-minded practitioner to be tentative in their own knowledge. In generating data in participative ways with users, research-minded practitioners, with an understanding of psychoanalysis, would not necessarily accept at face value what is presented to them. Neither, however, would they analyse such presentations within their own theoretical framework – as Freud would have done. They would explore their meaning with those who express them:

> psychoanalytic interpretations are neither true nor false; their justification lies entirely in their subjective significance for the patient, and whether for him they make sense, in that they present his experience to him in a new and revealing light (Yelloly, 1980: 160).

Marxist perspectives

Useful summaries of Marxism for social work readers have been provided by Corrigan and Leonard (1978); Howe (1987); Rojek, Peacock and Collins (1988); and Payne (1991). We have two main tasks here. Our first is to reflect upon Marxist approaches in the claims they make for their ways of knowing about the world. Our second is to consider the usefulness of Marxism for helping us to make judgements about the validity of knowledge, ours and that which others profess.

Marx claimed scientific status for his theory of historical materialism and his data about what he described as the dialectical relationship people have with the social world. By these terms, Marx meant that the social world can be understood as an external, objective reality created by people, subject to their influence and forces for change, but also oppressive of them. This making of our own history but not in a way of our choosing is the central dialectic of people's lives that generates contradictions and tensions to be exploited for study and change. So the method for studying the world is to act in it – the bringing together of theory and practice into praxis. This means that we can only make sense of practice by theoretically analysing it. At the same time, though, it is engagement with practice that provides opportunities to develop understandings, or theories, of it.

Again, as amongst psychoanalysts, so also amongst Marxists, there has been considerable debate about the scientific status of its knowledge. Some argue that it is best justified and legitimated by reference to its explanatory scientific method and the causal relationship it reveals between the 'economic infrastructure' and 'ideological superstructure'. Others place stress on the interpretive powers of Marxist theory and the ways in which it helps make sense of the processes through which people's subjective understandings of the world are formed. For Marx, it is experience and place in the economic system, the 'economic infrastructure', which determines our subjective ideas, thoughts, expectations and aspirations, the 'ideological superstructure'.

A brief summary of Marx's theory may help explain this further. Through capitalism, where the means of production are owned by those with capital, people become commodified as labour, alienated in their work. They are cogs in the capitalist machine, used and exploited by the owners of capital to generate profit. Some people, then, have common interests in that they sell their labour in return for wages. Others have in common their ownership of the means of production and their ability to benefit from the profit which accrues through the difference between people's wages and the value of what they produce. These fundamental divisions between people form classes. It is the relation of people to the means of production and their social class that determines their experience. For Marx, it is this experience that determines their consciousness. Thus how people understand the world relates to their class position within it.

Later Marxists broadened this economistic theorising to take account of other social structures that intermesh and reinforce economic structures to influence our thinking and ideas. Social arrangements, such as the family and education, ensure that people continue to be available to supply their labour, willingly and voluntarily. These 'apparatuses of the state' are developed to

ensure that people are fit and healthy, trained and educated, and
cared for/controlled in some way if, for some reason of age and/or
ability, they are no longer useful for production. Not only do these
structures provide services necessary for the capitalist machine, they
also serve the state ideologically. These ideological state apparatuses
such as the family, the school, the media and social work (Althusser,
1971), have a key role to play in influencing the way people think,
how they view the world, how they conceptualise their position
within it. Furthermore, people are in a dialectical relationship to
these structures. They have themselves created them. Indeed these
structures sometimes developed as a result of working class
demands upon the state. And yet they are experienced as external,
as other than created by people (Berger and Luckmann, 1971).
Structures, such as the family and education, are appreciated and
valued for what they provide but at the same time they are
repressive.

In social work, Marxist perspectives have offered a valuable
critique of individualistic approaches to practice that pathologise
the individual and the family, focusing on private troubles without
seeing these as expressions of public ills (Galper, 1975; Corrigan and
Leonard, 1978; Leonard, 1984). At the same time, attempts directly
to inform social work methodologies with Marxism are in danger of
advocating practice that negates personal distress and deals only
with the 'hard' issues.

An understanding of Marxism alerts the practitioner who is
research-minded to the need to be careful about accepting at face
value what is said, and how the world is presented. Data would be
understood not as factual and the whole truth, but as information
constructed ideologically in a class society. This would relate to all
kinds of data: data as in policy, in organisational norms, in practice
guidelines, in what managers say, what workers in other agencies
profess to know and what users express. Acknowledgement of our
dialectical relationship to social structures, such as the family, helps
to alert the research-minded practitioner to the contradictions and
tensions of people's lives and the ambivalence often found in our
thoughts and hopes. It would not be the role of the research-minded
practitioner to reinterpret and redefine what others say within their
own Marxist analysis. Rather, Marxism alerts the practitioner to
the problematic meaning of data and of people's lives. It provides
theoretical concepts and understandings that may inform their
practice and enable them to engage with others in the pursuit of
meaning.

Feminist perspectives

Feminists have addressed both the sexism of Freud and the neglect of gender by Marxists. They have constructed gender theoretically to make visible and analyse the position of men and women in our society. Fundamental to feminist thought, research and practice is the conceptualisation of patriarchy and patriarchal structures through which inequality between men and women is developed and maintained. Walby delineates these structures as paid work, housework, culture, sexuality, violence and the state (Walby, 1990). The contribution of feminism to social work theory and practice has been significant although relatively recent (Wilson, 1977; Finch and Groves, 1983; Brook and Davis, 1985; Dale and Foster, 1986; Hanmer and Statham, 1988; Dominelli and McLeod, 1989; Langan and Day, 1992). Again, our main task here is to examine the claims to valid knowledge made by feminists and to explore ways in which an understanding of feminism can help us to judge the validity of our own knowledge and understandings, and that of others.

There has been extensive epistemological debate about the nature of feminist enquiry and the validity of its knowledge. One view is that the validity of feminism comes through its correcting the omissions of other sexist theories and research. Women must be 'added in' for social theories and analyses of social data to make sense. Such knowledge, claim feminists, is bound to be more correct than knowledge which omits women. Thus, in social work, attention to gender has revealed that the majority of users, carers and social workers are women; that these roles are accorded relatively low status and reward in our society; and that often women have little choice but to accept these roles ascribed to them (Finch and Groves, 1983). Representation of the views of girls and women within the criminal justice system, and recognition of their experiences, has illuminated the very different meanings of criminality and different treatments/punishments accorded to men and women (Cain, 1989).

Another view is that feminism is more than simply adding women in: it is seeing and understanding the world from the perspective of women. Fundamental to the claims for validity of feminist knowledge is its recognition of patriarchy and its exposure of the gender bias of knowledge that emanates from theoretical approaches and research formulated and undertaken within patriarchal societies. Articulating and analysing the experiences of the less powerful in society reveals a more complete knowledge. It takes account of the subjective views and perceptions of those who are in this position, but who also have an understanding of the views and perceptions of those who are dominant. Nielsen presents what is known as the standpoint epistemology position within feminism:

> Briefly described, standpoint epistemology begins with the idea that less powerful members of society have the potential for a more complete view of social reality than others, precisely because of their disadvantaged position. That is, in order to survive (socially and sometimes physically), subordinate persons are attuned to or attentive to the perspective of the dominant class (for example, white, male, wealthy) as well as their own. This awareness gives them the potential for what Annas (1978) called 'double vision', or double consciousness – a knowledge, awareness of, and sensitivity to both the dominant world views of the society and their own minority (for example, female, black, poor) perspective. (Nielsen, 1990: 10)

Feminists have been critical of the methods of science. In its pursuit of objectivity and supposed neutrality, science has been conducted in such a way as to objectify 'the other'. Methods of feminist data collection and analysis, developed from an understanding of the personal as political, have emphasised the exploration of subjective experiences and understandings – of the researcher as well as the researched (Roberts, 1981; Stanley and Wise, 1983). Drawing on the experience of consciousness-raising groups, feminists suggest that this intersubjectivity between and amongst women is the most effective way to reveal and understand the meaning of women's experiences. This of course raises the question as to whether feminist research can only be done by women with women. This is both a methodological and an ethical issue. Methodologically, the concept and practice of intersubjectivity provides both an understanding of, and effective methods for, women engaging together to generate data. Ethically, feminist researchers have realised that a woman may divulge feelings and experiences to other women that otherwise one might expect to remain within her own confidence (Finch, 1984).

The construction of 'gender' as a theoretical category and, with it, masculinity and femininity, has provided the opportunity to reveal and analyse ways in which girls and women are told how to be in our society – a being of lesser status. This is done in such a way as to make it appear as natural: to do with being a woman per se rather than with being what a woman is expected to be in a patriarchal society. Perhaps no-one expresses this more vividly for social workers than Elizabeth Wilson:

> Feminism and socialism meet in the arena of the Welfare State, and the manipulations of the Welfare State offer a unique demonstration of how the State can prescribe what woman's consciousness should be . . . Woman is above all Mother, and with this vocation go all the virtues of femininity; submission, nurturance, passivity. The 'feminine' client of the social services waits patiently at clinics, social security offices and housing departments, to be ministered to sometimes by the paternal authority figure, doctor or civil servant, sometimes by the nurturant yet firm model of femininity provided by nurse or social worker; in either case she goes away to do as she has been told – to take the pills, to love the baby. (Wilson, 1977: 7–8)

Feminism has directly influenced social work practice in a number of different ways, depending on the particular perspective adopted. Radical feminism takes patriarchy and the oppression of women by men as fundamental. It has led to, for example, women-only services such as women's refuges and rape crisis centres, places where women may be safe from the violence of men and where they may, by sharing their experiences with other women, develop understandings in ways that do not provoke guilt and blame on their part. Socialist/Marxist feminists combine an analysis of patriarchy with one of capitalism to account for gender inequality. Social workers adopting this position have, for example, developed projects to improve the position of women's employment and projects to lessen the burden of unpaid, obligatory care. Liberal feminists focus on sexism and, provided that this is addressed and eradicated, existing social structures and processes are perceived as not particularly oppressive of women. Liberal feminist practitioners have pursued incremental changes to improve women's abilities to gain equality of access to economic or social goods. Black women have ensured that feminist analyses and practices take account of race as well as gender. They have been influential in contributing to the debate about the dubious notion of the essential woman and the need to acknowledge, in theory and in practice, that women differ from each other – depending not only on their race, but also their class, sexuality, age and (dis)ability. In social work, feminism informed with an understanding of race has enhanced understandings of the family by taking account of the experiences of black women. The family can be oppressive, but it can also provide an opportunity for resistance against racism (Carby, 1982; Lorde, 1984). The effects of immigration laws on separating members of families have been addressed by black workers (Mama, 1989). Stereotypical and pathological approaches to black families have been challenged as racist (Carby, 1982) and the disproportionate number of black children received into local authority care has been exposed (Dominelli, 1988). Black feminists have developed separate, more appropriate services for black women, such as black women's refuges (Dominelli, 1988; Mama, 1989; Dominelli and McLeod, 1989).

Research-minded practitioners with an understanding of feminism would be alert to the importance of ensuring that women are counted in and not just assumed to be like men. Here we are not arguing an essentialist position that would regard biological difference as significant. Rather we are saying that, in a gender-divided society, women's experiences are different from those of men. These experiences need to be made visible and understood. Adding women in would play a significant part in evaluating policies, organisational norms and practice guidelines.

The effect of social welfare policies, norms and practices in confirming and maintaining particular gendered positions for women as mothers, wives and carers would be analysed. The contradictions and tensions for women in handling their gendered experiences would be acknowledged. Research-minded practitioners would be able to recognise the contradictions for a woman in coping with the differences between what she knows she should be, how she should behave, what she should think and feel, how she should look and how things actually are for her. Fundamentally, research-minded practitioners would be aware of gender and the construction of their own understandings and experience through gender and that of others – managers, workers and clients.

Engaging with others intersubjectively, particularly with users, would need to be handled carefully for a number of reasons connected with the possibly inappropriate use of power. First, if the practitioner is a man working with a woman user (users usually are women), the sharing of experiences in this way might not be appropriate. Second, careful thought would need to be given by the woman practitioner to the context in which intersubjectivity is used. There are ethical issues involved in the sharing of experiences and understandings when the practitioner has statutory powers which she may use. In Chapter 6 we return to these issues in our consideration of ways in which the practitioner may engage with subjects to generate data. Where intersubjective methods do have a less unequivocal part to play in social work is in the sharing of understandings and meanings of situations already revealed. The research-minded practitioner would engage with others in processes of unravelling the meaning of women's experiences in a society in which we experience systematic, but often subtle, discrimination.

Combining perspectives

The three perspectives outlined are not necessarily mutually exclusive. For example, feminism has made great strides by not accepting as separate and distinct the personal and the social, psychoanalysis and Marxism. Rather than see these as competing perspectives, it is more valuable for the research-minded practitioner to regard them all as having something to offer. In reflecting on the range of theories, one of the first, and perhaps most important, lessons to be learnt is that theory is not the same as truth. Theories provide ways of understanding the world that will do – not that are right. Theories are always temporary and are held tentatively. They are 'good enough' understandings and explanations until better comes along. Herein lies a tension for the practitioner. Increasingly, with so much public doubt about the efficacy of social work, there is pressure on the practitioner to act with certainty. We have argued for the need of practitioners to be clear about what they are doing, their understanding of need, their purpose for intervening. It needs to be stated that clarity is not the same as certainty. Certainty in theory leads to dogma and blinkered practices. Clarity in theory opens it up for scrutiny, not only by yourself but also by others. Contrary to popular belief, research does not provide answers. Rather it ensures that questions are asked. The research-minded practitioner is one who is tentative, not sure.

The French Marxist, Louis Althusser, in order to distinguish scientific knowledge from ideology, claimed that the former is concerned with the analysis of theoretically constituted concepts whereas the latter takes for granted everyday concepts (Bocock, 1988). Another way of saying this is that, fundamental to the process of research, and that of the research-minded practitioner, is the theoretical analysis of concepts and, through this, the deconstruction of common sense terms, or: 'Theory must come partly from ideas outside daily practice, otherwise it would only be a simple reflection of that practice, but it must not be totally outside recognisable practice' (Payne, 1991: 208).

Thus, whereas the theoretically constituted concept for psycho-analytic study is the 'unconscious', for Marxist study it is 'modes of production' and 'social relations', for feminist study it is 'patriarchy' and 'gender'. So the research-minded practitioner would decon-struct, or analytically unpack, everyday and organisational routine meanings in order to reflect upon theoretically constituted concepts. We earlier gave the example of 'race'. Another example is the way in which Finch and Groves unpacked the concept 'community care'. This had come to be thought of in warm and glowing terms. Community and care are both 'good'- sounding words. And 'community care' was contrasted with the harshness of institutional care. No-one could be against 'community care'. There was no need for debate – until Finch and Groves unpacked the concept and, through careful analysis of practice, revealed that 'community care' actually meant unpaid obligatory care by women in the community (Finch and Groves, 1980). This construction of the concept has spawned numerous pieces of empirical research, publications, changes in social policy, carers groups and so on, carers involve-ment in community care planning and all the rest. It has provided a richness in practice.

This chapter has illustrated the importance of critical thinking with regard to epistemology and theory. This is as much a part of being research-minded as is the process of collecting data. Research, like practice, should not be a technical process: it is an intellectual, critical and creative one. In the next chapter we propose a value base for the research-minded practitioner. Trying to be anti-racist and anti-discriminatory, and being concerned with the empower-ment of disadvantaged and vulnerable peoples in our society, are fundamental to this value base. These values are in themselves in danger of becoming part of the 'commonsense' discourse of social work. They too can become only 'good' words. It is important that such values are adopted in a research-minded way: in a way that is concerned with constantly analysing the meaning and effect of the discourse. Only in this way can we ensure that our thinking and acting support resistance rather than simply enhance mechanisms of power.

3

The Purposes and Values of Research

Social work practice is, at any one time, a reflection of a particular set of assumptions about the causation of personal and social problems and the most effective responses to these. It relates to theories of the way society operates and tests those theories by acting on them (Kingsley, 1985). In Chapter 2, we explored theoretical perspectives on the ways in which subjective understandings of the world are shaped through experience and social context. Research has often felt irrelevant to the social work world because it has not allowed for subjectivity.

The epistemology and methodology of positivist research do not sit easily in the repertoire of the social welfare practitioner. Practice and positivist research are different orders of activity. The rigours of large-scale empirical studies require a longer time span and vaster scale of activity. The essential values of positivism, objectivity, neutrality and determinism are also at variance with the value base, and the purposeful and humble activities of social work practice. We have argued that there are approaches to research that are more compatible with ways of knowing in social work. Practitioners can employ these and develop a different relationship with research. They can own research and make it compatible with the values and processes of practice. New possibilities will then be opened up. New enthusiasm may be engendered for more acceptable forms of enquiry as inalienable parts of professional activity.

Value issues in research

Although positivism maintains a myth of the 'value-free ideal of scientific knowledge' (Fay, 1975: 13), all forms of research enquiry are inevitably value-laden. In positivist research, values that influence the definition of research problems, the design and conduct of the research and the interpretation of what is observed and heard remain implicit. This raises serious questions about the researcher as 'expert', about who controls the research and for whose benefit it is conducted. Getting behind some of these questions can, we suggest, lead to new solutions which will encourage practitioners to be less sceptical of research and be more ready to approach their practice in a research-minded way. Social workers have had little experience of research being used to serve purposes which they would support. They tend to experience it as researchers descending on them for poorly explained and unilateral reasons, or sending time-consuming and apparently irrelevant questionnaires. At the very best, they may have been fortunate enough to encounter researchers who valued their own views and involvement (Fisher, Marsh and Phillips, 1986; Hardiker, Exton and Barker, 1989). These experiences have been ones of greater co-operation between researchers and practitioners but have still separated research and practice.

Yet social workers do want to analyse critically their own practice, do want to question what works and why, do want to compare notes with other practitioners so as to become more effective. Practitioners do reject simplistic ways of viewing complex human interactions. They are also anxious to point out in their agencies and to government where there are areas of unmet need. A greater congruence between the values and purposes of research and those of practice would help to set disciplined enquiry at the service of refined and improved practice. This is not a simple matter of rejecting positivism. Other models of research can also be exploitative. The issues to be addressed go beyond the broad mode of research adopted, into matters of participation, partnership and empowerment.

Issues like ownership and assumed expertise need to be made explicit. It then becomes more possible for practitioners to make informed choices, not only whether to co-operate with research, but whether to apply its approaches in their own work. If practitioners are knowledgeable about the uses and abuses of research, they can stop themselves from being exploited by those who pursue and apply its findings inappropriately in welfare agencies.

Beyond this, they will also find that they already possess the understanding and many of the skills necessary to develop research in their own practice (Whitaker and Archer, 1989) and to share this with others. Forms of enquiry which take the strengths and the values of social welfare as a starting point can be utilised. Major potential can be released by practitioners having the knowledge and confidence to be research-minded. They already are knowledgeable about social welfare and are, or should be, committed to certain key values. Practitioners can develop expertise in being research-minded and this is fundamental in their work for empowerment. Carr and Kemmis, for example, argue for an educational science in which teachers become critical researchers with colleagues, pupils, parents and members of the community developing research as

> participatory and collaborative; it envisages a form of educational research which is conducted by those involved in education themselves. It takes a view of educational research as critical analysis directed at the transformation of educational practices, the educational understandings and educational values of those involved in the process, and the social and institutional structures which provide frameworks for their action. In this sense, a critical educational science is not research on or about education, it is research in and for education. (Carr and Kemmis, 1986: 156)

So the research-minded practitioner can participate with managers, colleagues, workers from other agencies, users and other members of the community 'in the tasks of critical analysis of their own situations with a view to transforming them in ways which will improve these situations' (Carr and Kemmis, 1986: 157).

A possible value base for practice and research

A statement of values for empowering practice has been proposed by Mullender and Ward (1991). We reproduce it here in a slightly adapted form to explore it as a potentially acceptable basis for the research-minded practitioner. Whilst all six of the values listed below are essential, the sixth is a sine qua non – a meta-principle without which the others cannot function.

1. We need to take a view of the people we work with which refuses to accept negative labels and recognises instead that all people have skills, understanding and ability.
2. People have rights, including the right to be heard and the right to control their own lives. It follows that people also have

rights to choose what kinds of intervention to accept in their lives, to define their own issues, and to take action on them.

3. The problems that service users face are complex and responses to them need to reflect this. People's problems can never by fully understood if they are seen solely as a result of personal inadequacies. Issues of oppression, social policy, the environment and the economy are, more often than not, and particularly in the lives of service users, major contributory forces. Practice should reflect this understanding.

4. Practice can effectively be built on the knowledge that people acting collectively can be powerful. People who lack power can gain it through working together in groups.

5. Practise what you preach. Methods of working must reflect non-elitist principles: practitioners do not 'lead' the group of service users, but facilitate its members in making decisions for themselves and in controlling whatever outcome ensues. Though special skills and knowledge are employed, these do not accord privilege and are not solely the province of the practitioners.

6. All our work must challenge oppression, whether by reason of race, gender, sexual orientation, age, class, (dis)ability or any other form of social differentiation upon which spurious notions of superiority and inferiority have historically been (and continue to be) built and kept in place by the exercise of power.

To emphasise, this sixth principle overarches all others. In the event of a clash between it and any other principle, it should take precedence. Thus, for example, the practitioner would not condone the rights referred to in the second principle being used in a way which is discriminatory or which oppresses others.

Principles 1 and 2

These principles recognise that all people have skills, understanding, abilities and rights. This means not allowing unknowing subjects to be exploited by, what may be theoretically flawed, expertise which 'dehumanises the individual by treating her as an object rather than as an active, choosing, responsible agent' (Pease, 1990: 3; see also Filstead, 1979). Stanley and Wise argue for 'a more humane, less "scientific" and patronizing approach than one which uses people's lives as merely research fodder' (Stanley and Wise, 1983: 84).

Assumed expertise can no longer be used to legitimate control over data and their analysis. Nor can it relegate others to a subordinate, unequal and less knowledgeable position (Oakley, 1981). Expertise is often illusory in any case, as highlighted by Huxley's high rate of detection of errors in quantitative social work research (Huxley, 1988). Expertise is kept in place by mystification (Wadsworth, 1982; 1984). It represents a way of exercising power over persons (Heron, 1981: 34) and, at worst, can become

another agent of authoritarian social control [if] knowledge and power are all on the side of the researchers and their political masters, and none is on the side of those who provide the data and are subject to its subsequent application. (Heron, 1981: 34)

Likewise, practitioners should find ways of sharing with others their theoretical perspectives and assumptions that influence the ways in which they understand, and take action in, the situations in which they are working. The approach of the research-minded practitioner must be to attempt to restore the humanity to subjects (Reason and Rowan, 1981) by recognising the many ways in which understanding human beings in a social world is quite unlike studying a chemical reaction in a test tube, or any other aspect of the natural world. People, for example, think and choose, whereas chemicals do not. As Filstead explains it:

In this paradigm individuals are conceptualized as active agents in constructing and making sense of the realities they encounter rather than responding in a robot-like fashion according to role expectations established by social structures . . . The qualitative paradigm also includes an assumption about the importance of understanding situations from the perspective of the participants in the situation. (Filstead, 1979: 36)

Participatory forms of research go further. They value not just the subjective experiences of those whose circumstances or behaviours are to be understood but their active contribution, acknowledging them as the true experts of the direct experience involved (Stanley and Wise, 1983). Such models replicate good practice in recognising service users as expert in their own problem and certainly about themselves (Smale and Statham, 1989: 8, emphasis removed). Feuerstein (1986), in writing about developing countries, sees the active involvement of people at community level as having a great deal to offer to any research or evaluation process. They already know the area, the people, the way they live, their feelings and aspirations, and what the research process will mean to them. People have a right to become knowing about their own lives. Archer and Whitaker (1989) have urged social workers to become directly engaged in formulating research purposes. Practitioners know so much, including what needs to be understood or evaluated in their particular setting (Archer and Whitaker, 1989: 29–30). They also stress that, where active collaboration in research design can inspire a sense of ownership,

> Practitioners think of things that persons without day-to-day experience of the job would not know or be able to think of, are more ready to give information and to implement findings, become more aware of what they already know and are using in their work, spread their learning and valuing of the research to managers and colleagues, and acquire new skills. (Archer and Whitaker, 1989: 37)

Principle 3

The involvement of practitioners or service users in being research-minded about practice might respect the letter but not necessarily the spirit of the practice principles we propose. Much activity which manifests itself as empowerment or as citizen democracy can, on closer analysis, be revealed as co-optation to preserve intact the status quo (Bachrach and Baratz, 1970; Lukes, 1974). Furthermore, participatory processes not grounded in a clear structural analysis can serve to reinforce existing inequalities on race, gender, class or other lines (Croft and Beresford, 1990). It is the values and the consequent style of working which make them empowering, not the techniques themselves. Calling a meeting of local women's groups to advise on a proposed initiative to address violence against women in the home may not necessarily take into consideration theory and empirical work relating to family ideology and masculinity in our society. In the absence of these, false solutions may be imposed and the holding of the meeting used to give apparent legitimacy.

The seeking out of people's views in participatory processes is not enough. The subjective experiences, attitudes and opinions of practitioners, users, managers and workers from other agencies need to be understood in their structural context. The participatory process of the research-minded practitioner is concerned with developing 'the capacity of individuals to reflect upon their own situations and change them through their own actions' (Carr and Kemmis, 1986: 130).

The role of critical research is to provide opportunity for all to question 'commonsense' notions and understand the pervasive relationship between the ideas we have, our understandings of the world, and existing structures and relations of power. Social work is concerned with values and meanings and has as its purpose social and personal change for justice, equality and well-being. It is essential in working towards the fulfilment of this purpose that practitioners understand the relationship between knowledge and power and work towards an emancipatory knowing, for themselves and for those with whom they work. 'A characterization of social life devoid of the subjective meaning of these events to the participants does violence to the image of man which portrays him as not only a reactor but a creator of his world' (Filstead, 1979: 36).

We can count the number of elderly people in a given geographical area using quantitative techniques. However the allocation of appropriate services to them depends on far more subtle notions of 'needs' and 'wants', as Croft and Beresford showed in recording old people's own opinions, judgements, experience and conclusions (Croft and Beresford, 1989: 29). These researchers gave elderly people a voice by recording their own words – their subjectivities. They also engaged in a process with the elderly people to interpret the meanings of these views together – critical subjectivities.

Principles 4 and 5

Practitioners can enable service users to become evaluators and researchers (Holman 1987; 1988) and to reflect critically on their own lives. Holman shows that people living in areas of social deprivation can undertake research and put it to their own uses: to win grants for voluntary organisations; to convince authorities that certain kinds of action or policy change are needed; to survey the relevance and preferred future development of a local community project. Research can be employed by users 'to shape services in the way they want, to express their needs and demands and to campaign for their purposes' (Holman, 1987: 162). This can only be achieved where they have power at every stage: 'over the questions which the research is to address, over the selection of participants, over the procedure to be used, and over the uses to which the research findings will be put' (Pease, 1990: 87). Special skills and knowledge of the research endeavour can be shared with service users. Some researchers have worked in this way: 'We do not see ourselves as "outside experts" but rather as people who are committed to the struggles we become involved in, usually with particular skills to offer' (Network of Labour Community Research and Resource Centres, 1982: 119). A specific example given by Holman is where

a small team agreed to help the Tenants Group by employing their research skills to try and produce incontrovertible evidence of the link between damp housing and ill-health so that the group could use it to put pressure on public authorities. (Holman, 1987: 675)

In research for social welfare, the research process should be accountable to those it most affects or whom it could most benefit in the pursuit of justice and equality. If this critical reference group (Wadsworth, 1984: 11) is not involved, the findings, in all probability, will represent the interests of those who commissioned the research and not those who will be expected to use any new or redesigned services. Research for social welfare:

names the people for whom it is directed; it analyses their suffering; it offers enlightenment to them about what their real needs and wants are; it demonstrates to them in what way their ideas about themselves are false and at the same time extracts from these false ideas implicit truths about them; it points to those inherently contradictory social conditions which both engender specific needs and make it impossible for them to be satisfied; it reveals the mechanisms in terms of which this process of oppression operates and, in the light of changing social conditions which it describes, it offers a mode of activity by which they can intervene in and change the social processes which are thwarting them. (Fay, 1975: 109)

Principle 6

Anti-oppressive principles are as crucial in research as in practice. This is not only a moral argument. It is also justified because false results will be obtained if no regard is paid to these issues. In the previous chapter we acknowledged the argument of feminist researchers that much is missed when women's experiences are not sought or listened to. They have also suggested that the views of the oppressed paint a fuller picture in that they take account of the perspectives of those who oppress them as well as their own. These researchers have demonstrated that the whole basis of research design must be altered to make this possible. Smith and Noble-Spruell, summarising other authors, state: 'Feminist research emphasises a non-exploitative relationship between researcher and researched which is based on collaboration, co-operation and mutual respect' (Smith and Noble-Spruell, 1986: 139).

As Stanley and Wise point out, the conceptual procedures, the methods of research, and the research models have all been provided by sexism (Stanley and Wise, 1983: 165). Women's experiences of their own lives, and of the social world they inhabit, need to be taken seriously. We need a research approach which includes women and is informed about the mechanisms that maintain the pervasiveness of gender inequality. Thus research for social welfare, for justice and equality, must be about women and aspects of their lives relegated to the private domain. And, as Duelli Klein demands, it must be *for* women: 'I define research for women as research that tries to take women's needs, interests and experiences into account and aims at being instrumental in improving women's lives in one way or another' (Duelli Klein, 1983: 90).

In Chapter 2, we explored ways in which feminism involves ways of knowing different from the androcentric norm. The conduct and ownership of the outcomes of research need to be placed in the hands of women. At the same time, we warned against the kind of woman-centred approach which has no regard for a theoretical and empirical analysis of structural inequalities. Sandra Harding cautions against research studies which place women on the agenda as victims:

> They tend to create the false impression that women have only been victims, that they have never successfully fought back, that women cannot be effective social agents on behalf of themselves or others. But the work of other feminist scholars and researchers tells us otherwise. Women have always resisted male domination. (Harding, 1987: 5)

And, crucially, women come only in different classes, races and cultures: there is no 'woman' and no 'woman's experience'. A

critical appraisal of the woman-centred call for more women to be
in management is provided by Everitt, who points out:

> To promote women into management does not necessarily bring
> a change in values and policies in the organisation. Women can
> share the same values as the men in management they replace.
> They can reinforce, or be used to reinforce, those values, policies
> and processes which maintain women as disadvantaged and
> oppressed in the public and private spheres. It is important to
> reflect critically not only on the politics of women who may be
> promoted into management but also on the political processes in
> organisations, mediated through gender, class, race and feminin-
> ity, that render some women powerful and others powerless.
> (Everitt, 1990: 140)

An analysis of structural and interpersonal oppression and social
change, beyond gender alone, is needed to ensure that some women
are not used in tokenistic ways to maintain the status quo. Women's
experiences and their place in society differ within social classes,
racial categories and cultures. Through racism, oppression is
experienced more acutely and harshly by women who are black.
An uncritical woman-centred approach will once again leave intact
the status quo with regard to race and class. Too often the
experiences and understandings of black people have been left out
of the account. For example, a study of domestic violence which
recommends the introduction of processes making it easier for
women to report incidents must take into account the different
position for black women, and black men, in relation to the police.
The possible reluctance of black women to report has to be
understood in the context of racism as well as sexism.

The interrelationship of different forms of oppression must be
recognised, so that, for example, understanding is not based purely
on white feminist paradigms:

> Generalisations are based on the experiences of dominant groups
> and the terms of debate, direction and worthwhileness of issues
> are set by white women. Black feminism and black women's
> political agendas are conspicuous by their absence. There is a
> tendency that those working on research projects will exclude
> areas of experience which are most difficult, most controversial
> and perhaps least familiar to them personally. (Ahmed, 1989: 19)

A similar analysis holds true of research involving disabled service users. Davis, for example, writes with anger about a planned piece of academic research into different perceptions and images of disability (Davis 1990: 15). No part of the disability movement had been involved in planning the project, despite the fact that the researchers professed an interest in concepts such as power and empowerment. Having regard for people with learning difficulties, Gosling (1990) calls for a process of empowerment of people with disabilities which includes giving service users information-gathering skills and influence over the evaluation of policies and service provision. For this to become a reality, she argues, language and conceptualisation themselves – which affect research as much as practice – need to change. This will involve a clear shift in the power balance:

Reality has been subtly redefined by the imposition of an alien language of terms and categories which has extended people's dependency even further – excluding them from honest dialogue and interpreting their lack of articulation as an inability to express any meaningful preference or choice. This language firmly places the disability within the individual. It shifts the buck from the truly disabling consequences of poverty, discrimination, unemployment and other social ills. It is a vocabulary of centralisation, containment and control. (Gosling, 1990: 1)

Writing from a black perspective, Dutt has indicated:

How you interpret findings of research and what you consider evidence depends on your starting point which in turn is governed by your values, beliefs and personal philosophy. A researcher's own value systems have an effect on the subject chosen for research and indeed the outcome of the research. (Dutt, 1990: 11)

Black writers increasingly point to the invisibility of the black population in mainstream research efforts (Ahmed, 1989) and in major enquiries into service provision such as the Griffiths Report (Dutt, 1989: 34). Research needs to combat institutional racism by measuring the take-up of and access to services and the levels of unmet need amongst black populations (Ahmed, 1989; Dillon, 1990; Ali, 1991). Neither research nor practice can progress unless this is done. As with all areas of oppression, the entire conceptual framework needs to shift and to build on direct experience:

> The problem . . . is endemic in the general production of knowledge. Writers (including the progressive ones) seem incapable of giving a real consideration to the structures of racial exploitation and experiences of black people. (Ahmed, 1989: 19)

One answer is to place the research tools in the hands of black practitioners and service users themselves. Ahmed calls for research objectives which will actually serve black people's interests. She recommends the use of black interviewers and consultants to improve the quality of information gathered and to press for action on the findings. She also strongly advocates the involvement of black communities in the research process. This must be more than tokenistic co-operation. It must ensure that the research avoids negative labels in its conceptualisation. It should facilitate the dissemination and application of findings. Such a contribution by black people in the community can be further valued through an 'exchange arrangement' such as offering training (Ahmed, 1989).

An understanding of sexuality is fundamental to social work. The pervasiveness of heterosexuality within organisations (Rafferty, 1991; Hearn and Parkin, 1987) and in work with users of social welfare services is increasingly visible. The criminal justice literature has well documented the ways in which women and girls are controlled through heterosexuality and femininity. In the introduction to the aptly named volume on girls and criminal justice, *Growing Up Good*, Cain explains its preoccupation with the sexuality of girls, recognising that everyone who comes into contact with girls, including other girls, seems to be preoccupied in just this way (Cain, 1989: 4) and heterosexuality is integral to the social control mechanisms of penal practices. Some girls and women resist, though with the risk of ending up in the social welfare systems as mad, angry, naughty or criminal. The practitioner who understands these processes, who understands

> the discourse of legitimate and illegitimate sexuality [may be able] to find ways to help girls to reach outside it and beyond it and to begin to imagine an alternative. We must find ways of creating spaces in which girls can start to think of themselves and who they might be in new and, hopefully, far more varied ways (a

moment's introspection might tell us that we all need that).
(Cain, 1989: 5)

Examples abound that demand critical scrutiny of the pervasiveness of heterosexuality in policies, practices and language. The relationship between domestic violence, child abuse and masculinity within heterosexuality cannot remain hidden. Evidence from practice and research shows that children and foster children of lesbian mothers are less likely to be sexually abused and damaged than those living in families with men (Hanscombe and Forster, 1982).

Our everyday language and concepts are not neutral. They represent a whole system of assumptions and limited definitions which derive from the world view of those with the power to control. Both practitioners and researchers need to make conscious choices whether to accept this world view or to question and challenge it. If we decide to challenge, then we need to form alliances with service users on whose direct experiences new definitions can be built.

The interdependence of value-based research and practice

A close consideration of values does, then, indicate a way forward for the research-minded practitioner. This depends on applying precisely those values which should be essential to practice: namely, the values of reciprocity, rights, empowerment and the challenging of all types of oppression. Thus research and practice can come closer together. Practice is enhanced by being subject to critical scrutiny. Research is enhanced by principles drawn from practice. Research-minded practitioners will not be won over by the trappings of legitimacy, prestige and funding of much, particularly positivist, research. They will be less open to being exploited by its top-down methods and outcomes, or conned by its worse manifestations: what Reason and Rowan call the dreadful rubbish that is sometimes put forward as scientific knowledge (Reason and Rowan, 1981: xii). They will be more likely to answer back with research formulations and explanations developed through debate with users and colleagues.

Good practice, research and theorising are interdependent. Research and theory must be grounded in practice. Practice has a greater chance of being effective if it is analysed through the application of theory and research, and, indeed, if it leads into the formulation of new theoretical concepts. We illustrate this two-way process with an example from groupwork. Groupworkers can inform their practice by reading the theory about group planning. At the same time, contemporary practice in social action and self-help has, itself, pushed beyond the bounds of conventional ideas and led to new theory building about a process of 'open planning' conducted by groupworker and potential group members together (Mullender and Ward, 1989). Such ground-breaking work frequently starts through a trial-and-error process, often because the values of practitioners are at odds with more traditional methods. If their experiments appear to be effective, practitioners will try working in the same way again and may tell others about it. They may reach the stage of writing a descriptive account of what they have done so that others can copy it. Though it begins to demystify and explain practice, this may still not be research but practice wisdom. It has not involved analysing why the new approach has worked, with the result that it can only be copied in a rather rigid way. It cannot be adapted to fit new situations or new practice dilemmas. Jeffs and Smith note this difference between recording and analysing practice, and point out that the former results only in a host of 'practical guides' based on folk wisdom and often little else (Jeffs and Smith 1987: 5). Mullender and Ward have contrasted this development of 'practice folklore' or 'commonsense' approaches to practice with the process of research which, they say, can

> analyse, evaluate and elaborate the folklore-based practice in the light of available ideas and knowledge, contributing to 'refined practice'. Instead of a disappearing circular process . . . we get one which is critical, constructive and developmental where practice and research interact with each other. (Mullender and Ward, 1988: 83)

What makes the difference, they suggest, is asking the question 'why' rather than being content with describing 'what' is done and 'how' it is achieved. Why has the practitioner worked in a particular way? Why was this particular piece of work successful?

Reflecting on this for research purposes we come up with questions. Why do some children become alienated and find ways not to go to school? Why is the privacy of one's own home the primary site for violence against women? Why are new purpose-built offices inaccessible to people in wheelchairs? Why are there proportionately more black people in prison than white? Why are there more men in prison than women? Why does the local newspaper write horror headlines about lesbian mothers? The researcher's and theoretician's main contribution is to ask the question 'why'. The contribution of research-minded practitioners is to ask this question and to provide an opportunity for those with whom they work to ask it, too, and to debate the answers.

Practitioners have a responsibility to pose this question to arrive at understandings of assumptions underlying the interventive process. What meaning does their work have for those it is intended to help? How might their work be improved? Why do people have negative experiences of social work? The 'why' question is crucial: the reason fundamentally relates to values. There is an inherent conservatism in asking only the 'what' and 'how' questions. These questions do not lead into any broader examination of why practice may need to change, for example, to take account of criticisms by women or black service users, or any examination of why social problems have arisen which now require intervention. To move straight from what appears to be wrong – for example, from an assessment that children are being inadequately cared for – to the established agency routines to tackle it can lead to unsatisfactory practice answers. There may be, for example, a tendency to put pressure on the children's mothers to give better care, without asking why they had been prevented from doing so in the first place. More effective intervention might be better geared to meeting the mothers' needs, for improved housing or a more realistic income, in order to help them meet the needs of their children. All capable practitioners know this, but in routine, everyday work, with its high caseloads, inadequate resources and low self- and public esteem, they may find it an uphill struggle to apply that knowledge to the cases in hand.

What practitioners do and how they do it are only part of the story. Why they do it, and why service users do or do not experience it as adequate and appropriate, are often much more interesting but require appropriate research strategies to ascertain. In order to reach conclusions about the reasons which lie behind actions, research methods are needed which can encompass values, experiences, processes and meanings. The research enterprise itself becomes different when it stems from an acknowledged value base which considers issues of equality and empowerment to be important.

Practice can be improved, too, by being imbued with clarity of thought, critical analysis and informed choice of approach. Both empowering practice and empowering research depend on being participatory, encouraging participants to 'own' the outcome by setting the goals and sharing in decisions about the most desirable process to be followed.

The types of practices we have described have also to be negotiated in the context of social welfare *organisations*. Participants include powerful people in hierarchical agencies. They address other constituencies in addition to the empowerment of people in vulnerable situations. How social welfare organisations can be research-minded, how they can develop critical cultures, has to be the subject for another book.

4

A Methodology for the Research-minded Practitioner

This chapter serves as a bridge between the first three chapters, which have been concerned with broad general themes and theoretical issues in research and practice, and the following chapters which focus on stages of the practice process: formulating the issues and preparation, groundwork and access; engaging with subjects to generate data; analysing practice data; and evaluating practice. Our intention now is to begin to develop a methodology for research-minded practice. We consider in this chapter particular aspects of research methodology, particularly those of participatory research, that may usefully inform the practice methodology of the research-minded practitioner.

We use the term 'methodology' to mean a theoretically informed framework that can be used to guide and analyse the practice process: in our case, practice that is research-minded. We only claim to make a beginning in the development of such a methodology. It would indeed be inconsistent of us, and an imposition on practice, if we were to present a methodology for practitioners. We hope, though, that we have been able to suggest ideas that practitioners may try out, test, experiment with, reject, fine-tune, reformulate in the true spirit of research-minded practice and critical enquiry.

The practitioner who is research-minded

Practitioners may engage with research in a variety of ways. Being research-minded may take many forms, depending on the practitioners, the organisation in which they are employed, the policy context and the particular problems and needs they are seeking to address. For the same practitioner the ways in which practice may be imbued with research will be different for distinct pieces of work.

To illustrate possibilities for working in a research-minded way:

● In being research-minded about constructing a social enquiry report on a woman charged with theft, the practitioner will have regard for:
  the range of possible sources of data;
  the processes through which data is constructed;
  access to data;
  confidentiality;
  the meaning of data to the client, the court, the probation service, possibly others such as the media;
  their analysis, relating them and their meaning to other theoretical and empirical material (such as the wealth of material that there is on gender and crime);
  the audience and its use.

● The research-minded practitioner engaging in groupwork with a multiracial group of girls may focus on encouraging and facilitating dialogue within the group. This might involve:
  agreeing in a participative way the purposes of the group;
  agreeing objectives and how these relate to overall purpose;
  agreeing on group activities and understanding the relation-ship between these and overall purpose;
  agreeing ways of communicating within the group;
  agreeing ways of documenting proceedings;
  developing understandings of differing perceptions of group participants;
  drawing on theoretical and empirical material on race, gender and sexuality to understand the different subjective views and experiences of participants;
  findings ways to evaluate the work of the group.

● A research-minded practitioner working with residents to develop a safer environment for children may encourage them to undertake a traffic survey to produce evidence in support of a request to the local authority to close off one of the streets for a play street. This would involve:
  developing with residents an understanding of power and decision-making processes in the local authority;

reflecting on the use that can be made of positivist research in supposedly technical-rational forms of bureaucracy;
sharing expertise and skills in sampling methodologies and methods;
agreeing ways to collect data;
analysing data and report writing.

The reader may well be thinking at this point that these examples merely illustrate good practice. Research-minded practice is good practice. Our argument to incorporate research into practice is not one which is made arrogantly: we do not seek to impose our ways of doing things as researchers onto the practices of practitioners. Rather, we have attended to examples of good practice, of studies that have been undertaken of the ways in which professionals think in action (Schon, 1983). We have borrowed from research methodology and debates to contribute to the development of a methodology for such practice. Quite rightly, many of the best practitioners have rejected research as elitist and as providing only 'technological fixes' which serve to depoliticise social issues while enhancing professional status. Our intention is to reclaim research for practitioners of social welfare before practitioners are completely claimed by the new cost-effective enterprises of welfare, ideologically imbued with New Right notions of family responsibility and individualism. Our task is to raise, as significant, 'the changing character of the situations of practice – the complexity, uncertainty, instability, uniqueness and value conflicts' (Schon, 1983: 14). Being research-minded would raise these as central to informed debate, dialogue between all involved in practice, between practitioners, managers, users and workers in other agencies. We use the term dialogue to mean informed reasoned argument and debate between people intent on engaging in relevant and critical discussion in order genuinely to understand. The aim of dialogue is to open up for examination assumptions, theories, observations and judgements.

Schon contrasts ways in which professionals think in action, what he calls 'reflection-in-action', with technical rationality. He traces the development of positivism and, with it, technical rationalism in our education and research institutions. He points to the divide between theory, research and action – practitioners being expected to have the skills to apply the theories developed by others. Practice that is not good practice develops when practitioners try to fit the situation they experience to such theory. Schon contrasts this with

the process of reflective thinking. First, Schon describes the process
of fitting practice to pre-existing and distinct theory:

> Many practitioners have adopted this response to the dilemma of
> rigour or relevance, cutting the practice situation to fit profes-
> sional knowledge. This they do in several ways. They may become
> selectively inattentive to data that fall outside their categories . . .
> Or they may try to force the situation into a mould which lends
> itself to the use of available techniques . . . or, more ominously,
> members of the helping professions may get rid of clients who
> resist professional help, relegating them to such categories as
> problem tenant or rebellious child. All such strategies carry a
> danger of misreading situations, or manipulating them, to serve
> the practitioner's interest in maintaining his confidence in his
> standard models and techniques. When people are involved in the
> situation, the practitioner may preserve his sense of expertise at
> his clients' expense. (Schon, 1983: 45)

Second, he contrasts this with the process of good practice where

> the practitioner allows himself to experience surprise, puzzlement,
> or confusion in a situation which he finds uncertain and unique.
> He reflects on the phenomena before him, and on the prior
> understandings which have been implicit in his behaviour. He
> carries out an experiment which serves to generate both a new
> understanding of the phenomena and a change in the situation.
> When someone reflects-in-action, he becomes a researcher in the
> practice context. He is not dependent on the categories of
> established theory and technique, but constructs a new theory
> of the unique case. His inquiry is not limited to a deliberation
> about means which depends on a prior agreement about ends. He
> does not keep means and ends separate, but defines them
> interactively as he frames a problematic situation. He does not
> separate thinking from doing, ratiocinating his way to a decision
> which he must later convert into action. Because his experiment-
> ing is a kind of action, implementation is built into his inquiry.
> (Schon, 1983: 68)

There are a range of possibilities for practice imbued with
research differing in the extent to which research and practice
become one:

● the practitioner who practises with a spirit of enquiry, thinking like a researcher: making explicit assumptions and theoretical perspectives; collecting and understanding data within these theoretical frameworks; further theorising through practice;
● the practitioner who plans and undertakes a small piece of research relevant to their practice;
● the practitioner who approaches their entire work as though it were a research project: thinking through theoretical perspectives; clarifying hypotheses; collecting, constructing and interpreting data; documenting practice; validating and developing theoretical perspectives;
● the practitioner who involves others in the organisation and in the team in the research process;
● the practitioner who involves users, engaging with them in an educative process to understand the meaning of social issues and personal problems, and the effectiveness of services.

Practitioners and researchers may be compared in the epistemological position they take. The 'expert' practitioner in the positivist paradigm objectifies clients and maintains a separation between practitioner and client in the same way as the positivist researcher relates to respondents. And just as there are practitioners who act pragmatically, adopting without question the status quo, there are also researchers who merely crunch numbers with little theoretical analysis. The researcher and practitioner we are trying to draw together in this book are those that adopt participatory methods of enquiry and practice.

The participatory model

The three illustrations of research-minded practice that we presented above illustrate not only different forms of practice but different ways of employing a variety of research approaches: positivist, interpretive, critical and feminist methodologies. Common to all examples is the responsibility the practitioner has to understand knowledge and its construction and to develop and share this knowledge with those with whom they work. That people have opportunity to understand the processes of knowledge production, the relationship between knowledge and power, and the skills to understand and have acknowledged their own experiences, perceptions and subjectivities, is fundamental to emancipatory we showed in Chapter 2). Such an understanding is important to open the gates both to consciousness and subjectivities and to decision-making arenas. Thus we suggest the participatory model of research as one which may provide the practitioner with a methodology for being research-minded in practice.

Being participatory does not mean favouring certain methods over others. From the examples it will be noted that a range of methods of data collection, construction and generation may be used yielding both quantitative and qualitative data. What is important is that the research-minded practitioner clarifies the purpose of the piece of work in which they are engaged and chooses methods that will most effectively achieve this purpose.

In Chapter 2, we suggested that an important element of being research-minded is to construct concepts theoretically, particularly those that have become everyday, taken-for-granted language. We illustrated this with reference to 'race', 'gender' and 'community care'. So, too, 'participation' must be constructed in order to be understood critically. Being participatory means adopting relationships with all involved in the piece of work to enable them to participate appropriately. But, as we pointed out in the previous chapter, this does not mean that participation becomes the purpose. Nor does it mean that everyone will always participate equally, or that every view counts. People will participate in a piece of work differently, depending on their responsibility and accountability for it. To encourage participatory processes with no regard for the processes of structural and interpersonal power is blatantly to disregard the overriding sixth principle: that is, that all our work must challenge oppression by reason of race, gender, sexual orientation, age, class, disability, or any other form of social differentiation. To illustrate: a possible reason to engage in a participative way with men who are violent is not to accord credibility to their behaviour, but to work with them to enable them to understand the construction of masculinity in our society and its effect on them and others; the airing of racist views amongst colleagues and workers from other agencies is not to accord them any validity but to place them on the agenda for understanding and deconstruction. To encourage people to participate in the management of a social programme without attending to who participates and who does not, who is prevented from participating and by what or by whom, whose views are not heard, is to replicate in the process of social welfare practice the very same inequalities that pervade our democratic society. The practitioner who is research-minded understands participation critically. This approach to the participatory method is sometimes referred to by others as 'critical' (Carr and Kemmis, 1986), sometimes as 'dialogical' (Gitlin and Smyth, 1989; Jeffs and Smith, 1990).

The model for the research-minded practitioner

In developing a model of the research-minded practitioner, we have first identified stages in the process of practice:

- formulating the issues and preparation, groundwork, and access,
- engaging with subjects to generate data,
- analysing data,
- evaluating practice.

Second, the aspects of practice to be addressed in each stage are:

- values
- ethics
- purposes
- communication
- roles
- skills.

Table 4.1 summarises this framework with stages in the process on the vertical axis and aspects to be addressed on the horizontal axis. It is presented in this way to help locate the important issues and principles contained within the model. The framework is not intended as a blueprint, but as a practice and analytical guide. We hope that the framework will facilitate exploration of research-minded practice by practitioners and that its content may become richer through this process.

Value base Values in social work are rooted in the historical, philosophical and policy traditions of the profession. These include certain beliefs in the individuality and integrity of each person, in the capacity for sociability, humanity and citizenship of every human being and in the role of the state as enabler rather than as social controller, coercive or humane. These values were explored in greater depth in Chapter 3 and are applied in terms of reciprocity,

58

Table 4.1

Research-minded practice	Themes		
Stages	Values	Ethics	Purposes
Formulating the issues	Reciprocity and participation in context; empowerment; locating the boundaries of feasible projects; identifying interests	Ownership and practice of values; openness; being explicit; active negotiation of grounded realities	Theoretical analysis of need; negotiating needs and service responses in context of; reciprocity; emancipation
Generating data	Empowerment; anti-oppressive practices; partnership; demystification	Rights; reciprocity; defining admissible knowledge; partners; community of inquirers	Asking 'why?'; 'in whose interests?'; variety of methods
Analysing data	Being tentative; co-producing meaning; questioning hierarchy of credibility	Judging the truth through rigour and openness	Making sense; reflexivity; being prepared to be surprised
Evaluation	Place value on activity; judge value against fundamental purpose; involve all parties	Overt/covert; confidentiality; do not let the one who pays the piper call the tune	Critical reflection of effectiveness of personal and professional practice in context; to develop 'good', not correct practice

Communication	Roles	Skills
Demystify; openness and sharing; negotiating permissions; setting boundaries on what is shared	Multi-role practitioner; partners; induction into the participatory user role	Sharing; reciprocity; honesty; sensitivity; engaging users in participation; team work; pacing and phasing
Engagement with people first; reaching out to disempowered people; redressing inequalities	Facilitator; involving others; intervening rather than detached; reflecting on the personal	Involving people in the process; listening; observing; recording; classifying; interpreting
Dialogue between all participants; recognising complexity in stressful situations	Educator; enabler; facilitator; engaging in conscientisation	Putting interpretations to the test; no perspective allowed to be sovereign
Dialogue; appropriate use of power	Engage in and facilitate dialogue; enabler; educator; change agent	Data collection; analysis; critical reflection; recording; report writing

rights, empowerment and the challenging of all forms of oppression. These together point to a developmental rather than institutional (needs-based) or residualist (last-resort) model of welfare. The developmental model is based upon certain democratic/socialist beliefs in which the state is given a positive role in reducing social inequalities. Within such a model, a central purpose of social work is to develop institutional means of representing the interests of underprivileged sections of the community. The hallmarks of this practice are positive discrimination, advocacy, community participation and empowerment.

Participatory research values are clearly consonant with developmental models of social work and welfare. But professional practice has to operate within less developmental structures. The welfare state is being fundamentally restructured. The frontiers of the state are being rolled back and priority is being given to the mixed economy of welfare, self-help and cost-effectiveness. The values expressed earlier are relevant as never before, but they have to be negotiated with an understanding of the context. The space available to empower vulnerable individuals, groups and communities may be harder to contrive. The potential for oppressive practices may be much greater. The bases for reciprocity are much more unequal. On the one hand, the challenges of the present age are greater than they ever were. On the other hand, prospects for developmental work may be miniscule, but, the research-minded practitioner can at least endeavour to expose pretence and coercive values. This must be done with systematic rigour rather than with, albeit justified, angry polemic. The non-reciprocal and exploitative nature of some research and some policies and practices (for example, needs surveys in relation to children in need, family support and community care services when there is no prospect of resources) should be exposed.

Ethics are the sets of moral principles which are held by members of a group. They represent the active ownership and practice of the values: empowerment, rights, reciprocity and positive discrimination. It is impossible for practitioners to adopt this ethical stance if their practice is based upon coercive social control structures or if they engage in professional contacts which disempower vulnerable people in the interests of their social protection. This must allow for the possibility that social control can be turned on its head to become social/personal change and that vulnerable people can be enabled to identify, share and develop conditions for their own social protection. These are the principles to be striven for even if the structural space available for their achievement may be limited. For many personal, social, political, and economic reasons, intended outcomes may not be achieved in practice and ethical positions may not always be held consistently. But the ethical stance of the research-minded practitioner requires explanations for this. For example, a schedule based upon racist and sexist assumptions may have been used to produce evidence of a mother's unsuitability to be restored to her children (Ahmed *et al.*, 1986). The social work practitioners involved may not be in a sufficiently powerful position to influence decisions made on the basis of such assessments. But many are in a position to question the basis of the assessment, drawing upon theoretical and empirical data. Practitioners may be able to ask the questions and offer alternative visions to promote dialogue with those in powerful positions of social control and the mother and her children. Being research-minded requires us to 'own' the results of our endeavours. It will not always be possible for practitioners to use techniques, methods and procedures of their own choosing. It will often be possible for them to make explicit the values underlying such activities and to share the consequences with everyone involved.

Research-minded practice is explicit about issues of ownership. One of the problems about positivism is that the research endeavour is mystified: esoteric skills and techniques serve the interests of the powerful. In positivist criminology, for example, there is a meshing of interests between scientism, consensus and determinism (Taylor, Walton and Young, 1973; 1975). This may be an inevitable process in advanced industrial societies where science serves the interests of the state and, therefore, of social control. Martin Nicolaus, in a speech to the 1968 convention of the American Sociological Association, vividly drew attention to the sociological researchers with their eyes 'turned downwards, and their palms upwards. Eyes down, to study the activities of the lower classes, of the subject population – those activities which created problems for the smooth exercise of governmental hegemony' (Nicolaus, 1972: 39). He asks us to imagine:

What if that machinery were reversed? What if the habits, problems, actions and decisions of the wealthy and powerful were daily scrutinized by a thousand systematic researchers, were hourly pried into, analysed, and cross-referenced, tabulated and published in a hundred inexpensive mass-circulation journals and

written so that even the fifteen-year-old high school drop-outs
could understand it and predict the actions of their parents'
landlord, manipulate and control him? (Nicolaus, 1972: 41)

Similarly, Foucault has understood social work as social control,
engaging in processes of categorisation of the powerless, as 'clients',
as 'deviants'. These categories become mechanisms of social control
in that they are accepted by the very people to whom they are
applied (Foucault, 1979; Weedon, 1987). If this is part of our
heritage, and continues to be so, the ethical implications of being
research-minded about practice need to be addressed.

If the purposes, processes and methods of research and practice
are not 'owned' by users, if users are not able to become knowledgeable, then rights and reciprocity are denied them. A minimalist
position for the research-minded practitioner is consciousness
raising about these issues. The processes of knowledge production
and the ways in which knowledge is used to maintain inequalities
need to be exposed. Research can be demystified. It is hoped that
the explorations in this book will provide some pointers to the
prospects for empowering practices which can be built up from such
awareness.

Whose lives are we talking about in social welfare? First and
foremost, we are talking about people, groups and communities,
who have been disadvantaged by combinations of personal, economic and social circumstances which bear upon their lives. These
circumstances range from specific problems (abuse, neglect, family
breakdown, disabilities, delinquency, homelessness, poverty) to the
ways these problems are defined, constructed and managed (deviance, stress, scapegoating, punishment, therapy). Practitioners
operate around this range, sometimes accepting the problem
definitions of social control, sometimes counteracting these, mostly
negotiating around them.

This is where the ethics of the research-minded practitioner are
relevant. Academic knowledge and methods can serve the interests
of the status quo, the powerful, at the expense of the rights and
powers of vulnerable and disadvantaged people. For example,
prediction scales for child abuse can be used to blame victims and
poverty indicators can serve to absolve the state from the consequences of discriminatory policies and practices.

What does ownership in participatory research actually imply?
Traditionally, it has meant that, at best, respondents in research
projects are sent a copy of the report and sometimes a copy of

interview transcripts. This is a very passive and limited form of ownership. Ownership in participatory research implies that research and practice subjects are actively engaged from the outset in defining the terms and conditions of the project. They will negotiate sponsorship, whether this lies with funding bodies or managers. Problem definitions will be shared; it will be impossible to consider research about predicting child abuse without sharing the political, legal, ethical, theoretical and practical implications of such a project. Various issues underlying sampling methods will be actively discussed and choices negotiated. Data collection instruments (questionnaires, interview and observation schedules, case studies, videos) will be explained in terms of rationale, feasibility and implications for genuine participation. There should be no reason for instruments to be tools to trap people. Similarly, methods of data collection and analysis will be explored jointly. Participants will be made aware of the assumptions underlying particular questions or probes and the implications of different responses.

The prescriptions of positivist research about not manufacturing data, not assuming the point of issue and not asking leading questions would take on quite different meanings. If participants 'own' every dimension of the research, there is nothing to be manufactured, the point at issue is understood so it cannot be assumed, and everyone knows where, how and why they are joining together on a particular journey. Finally, the results of any project are also 'owned'. Ideally this means that results become enlightenment contributing to human fulfilment and betterment, whether through increased understanding, resources or self-esteem.

These comments may provide guidelines for profoundly idiosyncratic and unethical practices. Just think for a moment about ways they may make people inappropriately aware that they are dying, at high risk of child abuse or offending, vulnerable to depression or homelessness, or not a high priority for services and resources. Such prospects indicate ways in which participatory research can only be undertaken under certain conditions, such as reciprocity, empowerment or anti-oppression: in other words, through a developmental mode of policy and practice. These conditions define the boundaries and purposes of legitimate endeavour. Such congruent possibilities are not always achievable. Therefore, if some of the values and ethics of participatory research are used to raise awareness in less developmental contexts, then this has to be undertaken in relation to the values and ethics of those other contexts. For example, if someone is dying in a context where the culture and structure is one of closed awareness, more open awareness must be negotiated, if at all, extremely carefully (Hardiker and Barker, 1981). Confidentiality takes on quite different meanings in participatory modes of research and practice. Confidentiality can be a very important safeguard of human freedoms and liberties, but it typically relates to relatively imbalanced power relationships. For example, the doctor, counsellor or lawyer own information about a client which is kept in trust and confidentially. To some extent, people do not fully know about or 'own' the use to which the professional puts this knowledge: the diagnosis of disease, the assessment of personal vulnerability, the indicator of culpability. It is easy to see why confidences must be kept in these circumstances, in order to protect clients from themselves and others.

But the stakes are different in more reciprocal relationships. Here the purposes of practitioners are to empower and to counteract oppression in the lives of people with whom they work. One of the most powerful instruments of oppression is the withholding of information from people. Such information may relate to knowledge about alternative resources and possibilities. It also refers to attitudes of superiority on the practitioner's part. The meaning of confidentiality in participatory projects takes on a different hue: to withhold information is certainly inadvisable. Confidential knowledge and understanding is shared between all participants in the kind of developmental projects being explored here. Ethics do not provide participatory researchers with safe hiding places, and ethical dilemmas are not solved by writing about them.

Participatory research, like other forms, is principled practice. The context of this practice perhaps legitimates and requires rather more explicit acknowledgement and ownership of principles about reciprocity, empowerment and anti-oppression than is either possible or appropriate under models of welfare other than developmental ones. We should allow for the possible conclusion that participatory research is not the appropriate mode in every circumstance for every issue.

Purposes   What are the purposes of participatory research? Firstly, purposes identify the commonalities between practice and research. Throughout the book we have acknowledged that many social workers have considered research to be antithetical to practice, the one being more theoretical and detached than the other. As Whitaker and Archer (1989) point out, though, commonalities pertain to problem formulation, data collection, intervention plans and activities, analysis, review and evaluation. In these there may be differences with respect to pacing, feedback and intervention roles. While it is relatively easy to see the commonalities in the processes of practice and research, the differences are greater in some modes of practice and research than others. For example, a user responding to a survey of consumer satisfaction in social services conducted in the positivist, social survey tradition will respond differently to a research interviewer than to a social worker undertaking compulsory interventions with respect to a family member. Anger and guilt may be expressed in both circumstances, but may be more freely expressed in a research interview than in an encounter with a social worker. The purposes and bases for reciprocity differ in the two contexts.

Therefore, secondly, common purposes can be located in the way that both participatory practice and research aim to empower respondents and to bring about positive change in their lives. The process of participation may itself be empowering and change-producing, whether this occurs through reflective consideration upon a social worker's observations about one's vulnerabilities or participation in a group research project exploring access issues.

Thirdly, positivist research instruments can be used for participatory purposes. For example, Hardiker, Exton and Barker (1989) conducted a relatively positivist feasibility study of policies and practices in preventive child care. During the course of that study, some of the social workers completed the semi-structured schedules in collaboration with their clients. This facilitated empowerment in both practice and research. Similarly, one social worker used the research instruments to explore service issues with clients from minority ethnic communities.

Methods have to be selected in relation to purposes. Nevertheless, the same methods may be used for conflicting purposes. For example, a questionnaire can be used for purposes of social control, social amelioration or empowerment. To what purposes it is put depends upon the values underlying the practice, the conduct of the inquiry and the use made of the findings. How many of us have responded to market research surveys without understanding the ways in which we are contributing to one person's profit and another person's exploitation? How many users have participated in academic research without being aware that their time and knowledge have been exploited and not enabled to see why the conditions of their lives have not been enhanced? These issues are incapable of final or full resolution, but consideration of purposes should maximise the possibilities for more ethical practices.

Communication   The language and practices of social controllers and practitioners often mystify people in vulnerable situations. It is easy to see, therefore, how the language and practice of positivist research mystifies social workers. Purposes, knowledge and skills are not shared because they are used as instruments of control, oppression and exclusion. The social institutions of complex societies (legal, political, economic, academic, professional) partly buttress social inequalities. One way in which they do this is by monopolising and pursuing esoteric knowledge and practices. This may be to the benefit of some vulnerable people in some circumstances, but the possibility has to be allowed for that it also disinherits and disenfranchises many others from the manifold resources which social progress has generated: education, health, employment, housing and income. Modern knowledge may also exclude significant groups of people from the opportunity to participate in their own society, or to address the alienating circumstances of their lives, whether these relate to poverty, disability, ageing, sexism, racism, or any other non-valued way of life. Participatory methods aim to demystify practice and research by being explicit about purposes, values, skills and knowledge. Making things explicit is part of the process of sharing, which in turn should empower participants by building up bases for reciprocity. Reciprocity occurs when goods, services, understandings, wisdom, vulnerabilities and gifts can be exchanged. One person's vulnerability can be exchanged for another person's capacities in one dimension and exchange can occur in the opposite direction in another dimension. How often have community development workers found that mothers who are vulnerable parents (as most parents are!) can contribute creatively to a neighbourhood group or social action project? These possibilities are not even envisaged in more coercive scenarios.

The language of Marxism, feminism and anti-racism may mystify just as powerfully as that of Social Darwinism, Freudianism, behaviourism, genericism and communitarianism. None of these languages needs to mystify or to generate oppressive practices if purposes, knowledge and skills are made to serve anti-oppressive practices. It is easy to say this, much more difficult to practice according to participatory principles. There are certain roles and skills available to make such promises possibilities.

Roles Most social workers are multi-role practitioners, ranging from assessor, therapist, enabler, counsellor, through to advocate, broker, mediator, then to educator, consultant, co-ordinator, planner and political adviser (Baker, 1976). The cluster of roles adopted varies in relation to the referral issue, agency policy, legislation and welfare context. For example, a welfare rights worker typically plays an advocate role, whereas a worker in an intake team is typically an assessor. Research is often seen as a specialist role in social work, often combined with planning and political lobbying. The theme of this book is that a research approach may be relevant to many roles, especially in work where developmental principles apply.

The research-minded practitioner adopts roles in relation to the purposes of the work being undertaken. The main task may be to undertake an assessment which involves the acquisition of information, the study of facts and feelings, the formulation of risks, needs and resources, goal-setting, plus various forms of intervention (Curnock and Hardiker, 1979). Within social control models, these activities may be undertaken in a relatively coercive way. In an expert professional approach the locus of knowledge, skills and power lies very much with and in the worker, the bases of sharing and participation being relatively unequal.

For example, an assessment of needs may be made as a last resort, in which services are provided on a principle of less eligibility, implying stigma. There will be many reasons to withhold information in these circumstances and the client may not be the major requester of the service. Precise rules and procedures for collating and producing data for a form require the worker to be very precise about the ways data are processed and people are categorised: deserving/undeserving, eligible/ineligible. Collating data on types of applicants and services provided might produce classifications implying pathology and experienced as mechanisms of control such as inadequate personality, dysfunctioning family, socially disorganised neighbourhood or remedial help. An assessment of needs is typically made within an expert professional model of service delivery in which practitioners use their skills and knowledge to construct needs on a scientific basis and according to an explicit value framework: coping and functioning, vulnerability and support networks, psychosocial transitions and packages of care. Knowledge and skills may be shared but not reciprocally and information may not be exchanged as an integral part of the whole process. Research in this model is often seen as a process whereby a practitioner uses a client to respond to a set of predetermined research instruments and excludes them from the stages of problem definition, data analysis and dissemination. The warnings of Nicolaus (1972) about research and of Foucault (1979) about social work referred to earlier may coalesce to strengthen professional intervention as a form of control. Practice imbued with research may thus negate the chances for emancipatory practice.

In participatory work, knowledge and skills will be shared reciprocally with a view to empowering consumers. Participatory models require practitioners and users to be role partners. The dynamics, status and obligations of most professionals as role incumbents indicate that most power and authority lies with and in them: assessor, enabler, broker, educator. In participatory models, these roles become activities to be shared reciprocally: assessing, enabling, educating. Practitioners will need to share understanding about role requirements, the bases of reciprocity and the meanings of empowerment and partnership.

Skills Social work skills are typically classified as: observing, listening, recording, informing, communicating, 'working with', pacing, liaising, representing. All these skills are also relevant in participatory research, their purpose being to empower all participants. Sharing and reciprocity may not be the typical expectations of participants in either a social work or a research project. There will be little room for building up credibility when the work is based upon coercive social control systems, since the 'user' does not particularly wish to be a recipient of the service. Even within a professional framework, credibility is seen to be more a property of the practitioner than of the user who is the recipient of the service.

One means of establishing credibility in participatory research is mutual identification of potential bases for reciprocity. We have argued that one person's vulnerability may be another person's strength and vice versa. This is surely a sound means of building up credibility. It still has to be negotiated in a skilled manner, otherwise some participants may feel patronised, devalued or trapped. Skills are required to identify and share issues and dilemmas and to use all one's antennae to listen, observe, pace and exchange information.

We have mapped out very broadly a methodology for the research-minded practitioner. Now our task is to begin to explore in more detail each stage of research-minded practice. In the next chapter we start with the stage concerned with formulating issues, preparation, groundwork and access.

5

Formulating the Issues in Research-minded Practice

Problem-definition and assessment is not a simple objective measure but a complex process which involves values, principles, agency policies and procedures, the current legal position and the perspectives of social workers and their managers. Similar situations may or may not lead a client to seek help, a social worker to open a case file, a court to make an order. (Hardiker, Exton and Barker, 1989: 112)

The idea of practice theory helps us to see that social workers are involved in an active process of conceptualisation in their day to day work; to describe this as the use of experience underestimates the similarities between the thought processes and conceptual struggles we engage in when we work with clients and when we read books . . . . The practice theories which social workers carry around in their heads, and which provide them with frameworks by which they can filter a mass of data, come from somewhere. (Curnock and Hardiker, 1979: 6)

The first of these quotations is from a research report commissioned by the Department of Health: the second originates from a book on practice theories. It is interesting in retrospect to reflect upon the similarities in the points made: this is the message we are trying to convey in this book. We are aiming to retrieve and to reclaim an intellectual tradition in social work by exploring some of the ways in which certain types of research methodologies can be used to develop social work practice methodologies.

We argued in the first chapter that research and practice in social work have developed in opposite directions, for a variety of reasons.

It is easy to see, then, why an objective and scientific approach to problem definitions and assessments (delinquency, schizophrenia, poverty, family dysfunction, child abuse) have developed in sharp contrast to practice ideas about vulnerability, stress, pain, loss and good enough parenting. The intellectual traditions, epistemologies, values and purposes of positivist research and practice wisdom have been quite distinct. It has been hard to see how research methodologies could be used to develop social work methodologies. In fact, not only has research done little to help practitioners, research has also been used to deskill and blame them for practising within the wrong (for example, unrigorous) frames of reference.

Problem definitions and assessments are complex and active processes of conceptualisation. There is a lot of territory to be unpacked if we are to trace this process, especially if this is to be put into service for practitioners. For example. pathways to welfare are multiple and contingent with many social, political, economic and psychological influences shaping decisions about accepting referrals and opening case files (Hardiker and Barker, 1986). Fundamentally, the practitioner who is research-minded will be aware of the problems in categorising client need and the organisational processes in framing and making responses to those categories. Being research-minded involves the critical scrutiny of what is often taken for granted, such as need definitions based upon behavioural, social or psychodynamic ideas, or agency filing systems which place people in administrative (statutory orders) rather than psychosocial categories (coping/functioning, vulnerability and good enough parenting).

The first quotation at the opening of this chapter illustrates some of the ways in which problem formulations in social work involve complex processes of social construction. Outcome is shaped by the values underlying welfare (needs or rights, social control or social change), agency functions, legislation and the orientations of workers. All these factors have a bearing upon client careers, on the ways in which potential clients think that the agency can offer them a service; the accessibility of the service, and the rules and procedures defining whether a service is offered and taken up.

Practitioners who are research-minded will have a broad perspective upon client careers. Not only will they understand the ways in which social work assessments involve negotiations about problem definitions, they will also think critically about the structures which shape the pattern of client careers.

In the organisation, for example, data may be collected to monitor the characteristics of referrals: address, referrer, social and demographic circumstances (age, sex, ethnicity) and initial referral problem. Many social services departments undertake monitoring exercises of this kind. But the research-minded practitioner will take the exercise further, incorporating research criteria and skills into the process. It is not easy to collect and collate this type of data. Every practitioner knows that, if the value of data is not recognised or utilised in the agency, then the process of form filling for statistical purposes can become ad hoc in the extreme. Practitioners will only record what appear to be relevant at the time. They will often make arbitrary decisions as to the category in which to place a client. If an agency is research-minded and data are used to facilitate informed dialogue within the agency, for example, through supervision, team meetings and working parties, then practitioners will take the exercise of form filling more seriously. Practitioners, with others as appropriate, need to be involved in the design of forms to ensure that they are structured adequately and appropriately to generate information that will be valuable to the processes of service design and delivery. For example, to ensure that services are appropriate for all, black and white, Ahmed has provided valuable guidance on the collection and analysis of data on ethnicity (Ahmed, 1989). Without such guidance from people who know, questions may be asked in racist and insensitive ways or may not be asked at all, leaving the services in a state of ethnocentric ignorance.

Being research-minded will also remind the practitioner to think about the implications of missing data. Certain vulnerabilities or agency responses may be unrecognised or screened out at various stages in the referral process. For example, people in one neighbourhood may have good access to packages of care because there is effective communication between the local health centre and the intake team. In contrast, another neighbourhood with similar needs may receive a low level of service provision, largely because referral points are inadequate. Thinking about missing data is a basic skill for the research-minded practitioner.

Being research-minded may well raise questions in relation to the careers of clients once they are accepted for a service. Patterns of case closure may illustrate dilemmas in service provision. For example, some critical questioning may show that people with learning difficulties are serviced routinely rather than professionally (Hardiker and Barker, 1981), that black offenders receive disproportionately high tariff sentences (Home Office, 1986) and that black children in care are rarely rehabilitated to their natural families (Ahmed *et al.*, 1986). Conversely, families assessed as of low risk and low need may receive services more appropriately directed to more disadvantaged communities.

These illustrations oversimplify complex social realities. They are introduced as a means of thinking about the links between research, practice and welfare objectives/methods in social work. In research, formulating the problems and issues to be addressed also includes processes of preparation, groundwork and access. A practitioner's response to us may well be that there is no time in practice to prepare, to do the groundwork, to think before acting. Our reply is threefold. First, that thinking and acting are not separate and the processes of both research and practice are not linear. Thoughts and acts proceed together, informing and influencing each other. Schon describes this process that is familiar to all of us: 'Phrases like "thinking on your feet", "keeping your wits about you", and "learning by doing" suggest not only that we can think about doing but that we can think about doing something while doing it' (Schon, 1983: 54).

At the same time, we would also argue that there has to be time sometimes to stand back, to plan, to anticipate, to question. Ten minutes before a groupwork session to clarify in your mind the purposes of your involvement in it may facilitate open discussion about purposes in the group. Schon points out:

> as practice becomes more repetitive and routine, and as knowing-in-practice becomes increasingly tacit and spontaneous, the practitioner may miss important opportunities to think about what he is doing . . . . And if he learns, as often happens, to be selectively inattentive to phenomena that do not fit the categories of his knowing-in-action, then he may suffer from boredom or burn-out and afflict his clients with the consequences of his narrowness and rigidity. (Schon, 1983: 61)

Our third point is that in good practice a lot of time is spent in groundwork and preparation anyway.

Being research-minded starts a long way back in the process, thinking fundamentally about the very nature of the project in which you are engaged. Any researcher knows what this means: read the literature, review existing evidence, develop a conceptual framework, think about the feasibility of different project designs, gain necessary permissions and so on. From our perspective, these tasks will be undertaken within a particular set of value premises whereby practitioners acknowledge themselves as an integral part of the process.

A first stage in preparation is to think about the general ethical, political and policy implications of the particular piece of work. The practitioner may be planning a piece of work in relation to service users or service providers at different levels in the organisation. The first issue to consider must be the purposes of the activity. These will shape the value frames and the boundaries of the project. The purposes of projects undertaken by practitioners who are research-minded may be broadly defined as passionate scholarship and social investigation which are put to use in the interests of personal/social amelioration and psychosocial functioning.

Value base

Empowerment implies that methodologies will not be used to disempower or alienate participants in the process. Empowerment must, however, be considered in its social contexts, as Sainsbury (1985; 1987) has argued so eloquently. For example, users' views on service provision and social work practice should never be used as a sole criterion of evaluation. Service providers have many other constituencies to address. And, as we have already argued in previous chapters, subjective views, including the views of users, need to be understood for their meaning and the ways in which they are shaped and given expression in our society. 'The success of research is rather to be found in the way it invades the thought-perspectives of staff and in the extent to which it generates interest in the possibility of co-research' (Sainsbury, 1987: 643). Empowerment in this context implies sharing, explanation, involvement, clarification and reciprocity from the very earliest stages in formulating issues.

The other side of the coin is to locate the boundaries of feasible projects. Research is always partial: so too is practice. Both can only ever offer a segmental perspective on or response to what is being addressed. During the preparation and groundwork stages, there will be discussions of influences on services and practices, such as law, resources, policies, organisations, professional values and ideologies and personal preferences. Unpacking and clarifying these respective influences should make clear proposed value bases and boundaries, basically the general, ethical, political and policy implications of the piece of work.

Problem formulation relates to patterns of service delivery as well as to the difficulties and circumstances of clients. The ways agencies define problems may close off services to some groups in need and give priority to other groups who could be offered more appropriate services elsewhere. For example, some social services departments explicitly define their primary prevention services as those which divert applicants to more universalist provisions or voluntary and informal support networks in the community (Hardiker, Exton and Barker, 1989).

The values of the research-minded practitioner indicate that consideration is given to the participatory interests involved. These are not confined to agencies and workers. This raises issues regarding who is the client, which in turn will be explored in terms of reciprocity, rights, empowerment and anti-oppression. For example, unitary perspectives invite wide consideration of a range of target and change-agent systems in addition to those of identified clients. This is an acceptable conceptualisation of participatory interests, but may lead to coercive practices unless the approach is understood theoretically and values implicit within these theories are addressed. Langan (1985), for example, analyses the value implications of systems theory which underpins the unitary approach. Social workers, intent on ensuring equilibrium in systems, may well coerce women to live harmoniously within oppressive domestic, caring and family arrangements (Langan, 1985).

Just because target or change-agent systems have been identified, it cannot be assumed that they are relevant participatory interests. The bases of reciprocity and participation have to be explored, otherwise the potential is created for coercive and disempowering practices. In practice that is research-minded, the process of formulating problems will not be assumed implicitly and imposed from above by the practitioner or agency. It will be a matter for informed dialogue on the basis of reciprocal explorations by all parties. This has to allow for the possibility that problems will be formulated which were previously invisible to the practitioner and the social welfare agency.

For example, a practitioner may wish to develop awareness of the levels of physical and sexual abuse experienced by adults with learning difficulties living in families or with other informal carers (Dunne and Power, 1990). Formulating the problem in this area is likely to be a veritable minefield: this may be why it is so rarely done. The practitioner may have direct or inferential evidence about the problem or may make some hypothetical deductions on the basis of her knowledge and experience. For, after all, if these forms of abuse exist in a patriarchal society and in family groupings which do not have disabled members, there is no reason to expect that some adults with learning difficulties are not abused. In many families, appropriate protective mechanisms operate, but sometimes circumstances induce or permit exploitation. The worker will also consider ways in which secrets operate more powerfully than usual in these situations. The process of problem formulation is just like research activity in this type of practice.

The practitioner will aim to engage with a variety of participants: carers, people with learning difficulties and other workers, say at day centres, or home care assistants. The problem will not be posed in terms of abuse (sexual or otherwise) but in relation to the rights and bases for reciprocity of all members of groups, and the ways these may be distorted, imbalanced or unprotected in families where there is a disabled member. Incestuous relationships may have a reciprocal dimension, but the bases of reciprocity are unacceptable. But to whom are they unacceptable? Values regarding anti-oppression and empowerment lead the worker to advocate for people in contexts of inequality: people with learning difficulties who are abused.

Clarity about value issues and value positions should help the practitioner who is research-minded to negotiate problem formulations in non-coercive ways. Social workers should never accept the problem definitions of others without reformulating them. This involves consideration of, and negotiation with, a wide variety of participants both in the client's community and in welfare agencies. We now turn to consideration of some ethical issues.

Ethics

Rights, reciprocity, empowerment and anti-oppression can be formulated as ethical principles to underpin practices. If social worker–client relations are reciprocal, these will form an active part of the process of problem formulation. This is typically seen in terms of identifying clients' rights and oppressions with a view to creating new opportunities for reciprocity and empowerment. The other side of the coin, though, is to negotiate the boundaries and potential for manageable projects: neither social workers nor clients are free-floating participants in the process. Problem formulation is not a purely abstract exercise but the active negotiation of grounded realities.

For example, a group of welfare workers from a variety of agencies and also black parents may be concerned about the needs of black children in care. Preliminary concerns include the disproportionate numbers of black children in care, the scale of drift, possibilities of cultural genocide and racism. How does one begin to locate a manageable project in these circumstances?

● First, political implications are considered. Is the concern legitimate? This can be contextualised in relation to equal opportunities and race relations legislation together with the provision about taking children's social and cultural circumstances into consideration in the 1989 Children Act.

● Second, local authority policies in respect of equal opportunities will have a bearing in this area. Even so, the focus of these anti-discriminatory policies may be assimilationist or integrationist. As such, they may not recognise the value of culture and the racist mechanisms that impose certain white cultures upon others.

● Third, the agency and resource context is relevant. Do workers and parents have legitimate access to the decision makers who are part of the discrimination process in children's services? The careers of children in care are influenced by a wide range of people, from those in control of, say, education, health, law, social services and voluntary agencies, to lay referrers such as neighbours, kin, friends or enemies.

Many professional, academic and voluntary groups have, of course, actively campaigned for black children in care. Are we merely suggesting ways of joining this stream? To some extent we are, but we are also arguing that a research focus can enable practitioners to incorporate these concerns as an integral part of their social work practice. Using one's values, knowledge and skills to lay bare the choices and to identify the permeable boundaries of legitimate endeavour should always be part of the repertoire of the practitioner. This is crucial at the problem-formulation stage and in preparation and groundwork for a piece of work (Hardiker and Barker, 1991).

One approach to bounding and widening the problem-formulation stage might be to hold a conference. The main aim of the conference would be to solicit a wide range of views from legitimate interests and to construct a feasible formulation of the problem. The structures and functions of agencies which resource legitimate endeavour would be examined. Ethical imperatives indicate the inappropriateness of promising much and providing little. Data on black children in care should not be collected if they are not going to be used. Black interests will be actively informed about the basis of their participation and their knowledge and understanding built into the processes.

Such a project is manifestly ambitious, but built into it from the outset are structures which permit participants to withdraw and to decide that they do not wish the project to proceed. If the bases of rights and reciprocity are actively addressed and met, withdrawal will be a proactive and empowering process rather than an embittered, reactive or coercive one. Pointers to alternative problem formulations may be rehearsed and other channels of influence or change identified.

Ethical work builds in consideration of manageable projects from the outset of any piece of work. This locates both the boundaries and the prospects of legitimate endeavour. The assumption is that knowledge and understanding about obstacles to activity can be as empowering as guidelines and support.

Purposes

When formulating problems, the research-minded practitioner will locate purposes which are concerned with theoretical reflection and analysis as well as with meeting needs and providing services. Reciprocity and empowerment are fundamental to both. Theorising through practice is undertaken with all participants and is undertaken in such a way as to enhance the capacity of all to learn through experience.

Identifying the boundaries of acceptable practice involves consideration of unacceptable purposes. Developing a trained incapacity to rise above a series of cases is not part of the purposes of the research-minded practitioner. Research-minded practitioners will always work with 'cases' in terms of public issues as well as private troubles (Mills, 1959), recognising that social and interpersonal oppression is experienced in feelings of distress and anguish. Using clients merely as a source of data is not an acceptable project. Their valued resources must be strengthened and they must be provided with opportunities to be more knowledgeable and understanding of the lives they lead and to use their evidence to mobilise better services. Anti-oppressive practices imply that, in being research-minded, practitioners engage in non-exploitative and potentially emancipatory relationships at every stage of their work.

The purposes of problem formulation are to explore and negotiate ways in which users and potential users of services and practitioners can define needs in ways which agencies can address. This has also been a hallmark of more traditional work, in which referrals are negotiated in relation to agency functions. The research-minded practitioner will adopt a broad perspective towards this task. We have argued that agency categories of need will not be used rigidly and the possibility of developing different need classifications will always be considered. For example, the social dimensions of health and development in the Children Act regarding children 'in need' will be actively constructed in terms of social deprivation as well as vulnerable families (In Need Implementation Group, 1991). Evidence will be collated on need definitions with a view to developing a more population-based rather than individualised response to service delivery.

Purposes are thus always conceptualised broadly but still grounded firmly in the realities of the political economy of social work practice. Problems are never reformulated in ways which are divorced from service delivery and client empowerment; research-minded practitioners never engage in indulgent exercises which merely lead to their own self-aggrandisement.

Recognition will be given to the fact that people have privacy and own information about themselves and others. Some people in our society are allowed more privacy than others. One only has to reflect on the many studies of people in poverty compared with the few on the wealthy. Doors without long drives leading up to them are easier to knock on! People as users of social services should be aware that they have rights with regard to the disclosure of information. They should know why they are telling what, to whom such information will then be available and what the consequences are or may be for them and others. The process of formulating problems always involves reciprocal relations, in which practitioners aim to enhance clients' rights and strengthen their capacities and their potential for sociability in civil society.

Communication

So far we have been making some rather grandiose claims about the processes involved in formulating problems. The claims are less grandiose if they are firmly grounded in the realities of social work, welfare and political economy. The structures and processes of these realities need to be understood thoroughly if the practitioner is to communicate in non-oppressive ways with all participants in the process.

Interpreting the nature of the project is a skilled and complex task, given that many participants are vulnerable because of their many and enduring experiences of loss, hardship and discrimination. Why should they offer their perspectives on and understandings of their problems, if their life experiences have taught them the bitter costs of such disclosure: a child taken into care, a spouse imprisoned, a relative removed under a psychiatric order? This obviously represents the sharp social control dimension of social work practice, but it has to be thoroughly understood by research-minded practitioners who will have to communicate their purposes skilfully.

For example, a practitioner may plan to find ways to take account of the experiences of parents whose children have been admitted to care. Through the 'repertoire of examples, images, understandings and actions' (Schon, 1983: 138) built up over years, the practitioner has concerns that the experience for parents is one of coercion. Her intentions are to develop ways to make this experience more understandable to those keenly involved. Collating parents' views will mean the practitioner addressing their anger, loss, hopes and bitterness. Controlling catharsis, aggression and depression will also be necessary. Staying with these transactions while formulating a basis for agreed work and more acceptable priorities will also require skills in communication: listening, observing, pacing, resourcing, liaising, mirroring and interpreting. Practitioners, in a research-minded way, will also use their antennae to think in terms of populations and vulnerabilities instead of individuals and deviance. Ways of improving services and their delivery across a wide spectrum of agencies and decision-making forums will also be incorporated into the problem-formulation stage.

The essential thing to communicate at this stage is the need to achieve some reciprocal agreements about the nature of the project: the topic, the boundaries of permitted and required endeavour and the methods upon which the work will proceed, including rules for participation and reciprocity. Communication will be open and shared because power lies with the participants in interaction with one another rather than with a professional imposing his or her will upon clients.

Roles

It has always been recognised in social work that induction into the client role is an important part of the process (Hardiker and Barker, 1986). Such induction comes into high profile at the preparation, groundwork and problem-formulation stages. Users need to learn about the rules of engagement, including what they will be expected to disclose and what type of services are likely to be offered.

Role induction is also important in more participatory work, since many users may not have entered into this type of role relation before. It is not necessarily clear or self-evident what rights, empowerment, reciprocity and anti-oppressive practices mean or imply. Users are not necessarily aware of the resources and strengths which they bring to a situation which involves a need or request for services.

For example, a practitioner may be concerned about the services made available to people with disabilities in a particular locality. Preliminary exploration indicates that the agency is inaccessible for a variety of reasons: physical obstacles in the building, transport difficulties, inhospitable reception facilities, a routinised referral system, social worker's ideologies which construct disabilities in narrow and pathological terms, unimaginative packages of care and superficial monitoring and evaluation. One practitioner cannot undertake to turn around such a large and complex service delivery system. What research-minded practitioners can initiate, if they incorporate research approaches into their practices, is a process whereby problems are reformulated by all potential participants.

A necessary part of the process of problem reformulation in relation to disabilities is to begin to work with participants as partners. People's experience of disabilities equips them with profound knowledge about physical obstacles, stigma, patronising services, routine processing, case closure before needs have been met, lack of consultation and pathologising problem definitions. The research-minded practitioner will think beyond agency-determined problem definitions and be able to explore alternative perspectives, such as social and psychosocial models of disability

(Oliver, 1983; 1989). These will be based on theoretical knowledge and also on affirmative values. They will highlight ways in which people with disabilities often lose their rights, fail to have their needs even addressed, are made powerless, particularly in the most vulnerable dimensions of their lives, and are rarely invited to engage in reciprocal relations. Whether experienced singly or cumulatively, these are extremely oppressive phenomena.

Therefore engaging people with disabilities as partners in joint processes of education is the basis for roles in problem formulations. The practitioner has skills and knowledge to share and has much to learn from such partnerships. Again, rules for bounding the project will be actively incorporated into these role relationships.

Skills

Once the topic and participants in a piece of work have been identified and located, the skill lies in engaging their participation. Why should anyone join in either a practice or a research project, especially if their past experiences of the same have been exploitative and oppressive?

Some credibility will already have been established during the preparation and groundwork stages. The same now has to be negotiated as the problem begins to be formulated. Negotiation implies that client participants have a stake in the problem definition, which will not be imposed upon them. Negotiation will imply that the practitioner not only shares the grounds of participation, but also illustrates what these may mean and imply.

For example, a social worker may be concerned about the ways female offenders are supervised in a probation agency. An examination of records suggests that the problems of these clients are typically individualised inappropriately in relation to their gender roles, such as parenting difficulties, domestic work and marital relations. These, of course, may be the major concerns of these women. Nevertheless, if opportunities are made available for both alternative problem definitions and different service and resource options, a less gender-oppressive provision may be possible.

The research-minded practitioner will be aware that the content of agency records may not accurately reflect the nature of the practice. The practice may be accounted for in gender-stereotypical ways, but be undertaken in terms of consciousness-raising and less oppressive role alternatives, such as waged work, community participation, other activities besides parenting and conjugal roles, and alternative self-concepts. The point of this example is that research and practice skills are brought together to negotiate the nature of the problem. Practitioners who are research-minded are not naive, nor do they impose their preferences arrogantly and without permission upon others.

Skills in negotiating with colleagues will also be required. By what authority does the practitioner plan to redefine a problem or plan of action? Establishing credibility with colleagues, as any student or new worker knows, is of the utmost importance. The creation of a community of inquirers which includes users, managers, practitioners and their colleagues and workers from other agencies would be the aim for any piece of research-minded practice. We borrow the term community of inquirers from Scheffler (1982). He describes it as a coming together of those participating in the project with everyone having 'responsibility to the evidence, openness to argument, commitment to publication, loyalty to logic, and an admission, in principle, that one may turn out to be wrong' (Scheffler, 1982).

Providing a less individualised mode of service delivery often points to the appropriateness of group work or similar projects. Anticipating this is itself incorporated into the problem formulation stage, since a group response may encourage a group problem definition.

Pacing and phasing in planning new initiatives are also essential skills. Otherwise this type of research-minded practice will be experienced in quite as alienating a way as some more positivist-inspired projects. The key to problem formulation is skilled negotiation around promises, boundaries and possibilities. However well these are jointly explored between participants on a reciprocal basis, the practice must be grounded in relation to the political economy of welfare practices. To promise much and offer little is not a skill, nor is it ethical practice.

A rather individualistic picture of the research-minded practitioner has been presented in this chapter. No practitioner is able to think whatever thoughts or to engage in whatever practices she pleases, even when operating within a participatory context. Consideration must be given to team work, to collective responsibility, to hierarchies, to legitimate authority and to the resources provided to sanction any practices. As this book is not about welfare organisations, nor even about research-minded organisations, we have not given a high profile to the methodologies required in relation to groups and agencies. This is a limitation. If research-minded practitioners are to work towards bringing about change in ways we have described, then the same values, knowledge and skills must be used as they negotiate with colleagues and managers within their organisations.

In the next chapter we examine some of the ways in which the values, knowledge and skills used in formulating issues can also be developed in participatory modes for generating data.

6

Engaging with Subjects to Generate Data

I am looking for something. Much of it is hidden and hard to find. Much of it is complex and slippery; once found it is hard to hold. I am looking for that elusive quality called experience. But how am I to find it? (O'Hagan, 1986: 2)

The popular image of data is probably columns of figures or piles of completed questionnaires. Data generation and gathering become far more complex than this as soon as value issues come into play. Subsumed within questions about data we find ones such as who generates the information? from whom? on whose behalf? and for whose use?

The word 'data' is actually the plural of 'datum': latin for 'given'. 'Given' these pieces of information, we can deduce that . . . In other words, data are the building-blocks for knowing and findings arise from manipulating them in various ways. But, in the process of acquiring these building-blocks – these 'givens' – who is actually giving what to whom, and do they understand the full implications? Social workers know, perhaps better than anyone, that there are ethical issues involved in the acts of giving and receiving. The research-minded practitioner will be fully aware of these and will be concerned to engage dialogically with others to generate mutually beneficial data.

Providers and users of data must agree on what counts as admissible knowledge. This extends far beyond columns of figures and questionnaire responses and is, in fact, an open-ended question. Different forms of data have their advantages and disadvantages. They also involve differing problems and dilemmas in collection and recording, which we shall examine here.   In the model of practice we propose, all participants are recognised as members of the 'community of inquirers': generating data, and having skills in selecting, accessing, prioritising and synthesising data.

Value base

One key to practice that is research-minded practice is its anti-oppressive value base. These values have been shown in Chapter 3 to be fundamental to practice. Consequently, social workers who have their practice well sorted out will have a head start in appreciating good research, whether they intend to conduct it themselves, to understand what it can achieve, how it can be applied to improve practice and what its limitations are, or generally to benefit from the rigour of thought in being research-minded.

The application of demystified and value-impregnated research skills should become an integral part of the social work task and can certainly enable practice to be developed in a more systematic way. It can help practitioners to make their concepts and assumptions clearer, to be readier to evaluate their own practice, to analyse critically the work of their agencies, and to do all this in partnership with service users. Establishing a value-based partnership has to be seen against a background of ethical considerations and concerns.

Ethics

Interaction between research-minded participants in practice must be framed by ethics of rights, reciprocity, empowerment and anti-oppression. We shall consider each in turn. Active involvement includes the process of defining what counts as admissible knowledge. An example may be taken from a study of law teaching in practice placements (Hogg *et al.*, 1990: 15). Here practice teachers and social work students expressed and reviewed their own ideas on issues raised by the need to know and use the law in social work. For them, practice was infused with all kinds of legal definitions, requirements and processes. This contrasts with earlier studies (Ball *et al.*, 1988; Vernon *et al.*, 1990) which have tended to work from the premise that there is a straightforward body of law that can be identified by those outside practice that the student either knows or does not know. No doubt most experienced social workers would agree that the application of the law in practice is infinitely more complex than this. It behoves research-minded practitioners to do all they can to reflect that complexity. If they fail to do so, understandings will be limited. In the example of applying law to practice the problem may not simply be faulty teaching and inadequate learning of rote facts (as has been suggested) but rather the need for a new conceptualisation of practice, the law and legal thinking.

In the previous chapter we noted that participatory approaches require that those involved in the piece of work know what they are getting into and are able to decide whether to opt in or out. All those with whom the research-minded practitioner works in the process of practice should be aware of the critical reflective approach that is being adopted.

This gives rise to a range of dilemmas. First, how far will revealing the research approach to practice affect that practice (Shipman, 1988)? Will other participants in the process respond to the increased attention, thus creating a 'Hawthorne effect'? This is named after the General Electric Company works in Chicago where this impact of research was first recognised (see Shipman, 1988). In a piece of research, this effect may well affect the validity of the findings. In other words, the findings may not represent the reality of the situation but rather the situation affected by being researched. In seeking to develop research-mindedness in practice, this effect may well have positive results. Knowing that you are to be critically reflective in your practice may encourage those with whom you work to be so as well. Or it may have negative effects leading others to cover up and be defensive.

Second, do all participants have equal rights to be informed about the research-minded process? We have already suggested in Chapter 4 that participation has to be understood in the context of power relations. The participatory research idea that everyone be fully included throughout the research process, and not merely used to provide data for the researchers, derives from experiences of research in which the researcher is more powerful than the researched: the experiences we referred to in Chapter 4 of the sociologist looking down to study the activities of the lower classes (Nicolaus, 1972). But there may well be situations in which research-minded practitioners wish to reflect critically on the practices of those more powerful than themselves. In her study of prostitution as an institution, as distinct from prostitutes, Smart reflects on such power relations in the research process. She researches the "locally powerful" – magistrates, local businessmen and employers or their wives (Smart, 1988: 42). In considering the ethics of her work, she comes to the conclusion that the feminist ethic of sharing the research purposes and data with those studied

> do not help a feminist who is doing research on the locally powerful who are predominantly men. Arguably it is important for feminists to study upwards rather than sideways or more traditionally downwards toward the disadvantaged. But if we do, we find that the new tenets of research do not help us a great deal. For example the basic assumption that the researcher is in a more powerful position than the researched does not always hold good when the researcher is a woman and the researched are well-established and frequently, in their own terms, important men. Such people are not afraid to refuse to answer questions to tell you what they think of your research, or ultimately to terminate the interview at their convenience. (Smart, 1988: 42–3).

Research-minded practitioners, critically reflecting on the practice of social welfare, may well be less powerful, both in themselves and in their emancipatory ideas, in organisations and contexts which are fundamentally sexist, heterosexist and racist. As Smart says: 'making ourselves even more vulnerable by discussing our reasoning and purposes to those we research is not *always* a useful policy' (Smart, 1988: 43).

Ethics should not be accepted as positivist facts. They must be contextualised and theorised. This holds equally true for what we now go on to say about the need to take account of all perspectives, all views. Not every view can be afforded credibility by the research-minded practitioner accountable to the values presented in Chapter 3. Views are shaped through processes and structures in a society divided by gender, race, class, sexuality and age. They are expressed by the powerful and through institutions to maintain the status quo, to maintain inequality.

So, too, research-minded practitioners will recognise that their own views are shaped and will be prepared to put them to the test. We see the world through our own lenses. In a dialogical relationship, it is better, wherever possible, to feed back what has been observed to those directly involved, to see if it rings true for them (for example, Fisher *et al.*, 1986: 31–2, writing about an attempt to treat the 'subjects' as co-researchers by using of this process). Everyone has their own biases. If a 'community of inquirers' exists, differences in perspectives can be discussed and understood. Differences may be ironed out. They may be reflected upon and new understandings reached. The texture of the account will be all the richer if different perspectives are included and theorised. Reciprocity implies a process of levelling out and an eschewing of the old hierarchies. The view from above must be replaced by the view from below. This means critically reflecting upon the powerful – people, processes, institutions and structures. It also means engaging with those often excluded from the processes of 'knowledge making' about our social world and according them credibility. This is the necessary consequence of the demands of conscious partiality and reciprocity (Mies, 1983).

> the way of co-operative inquiry – is for the researcher to interact with the subjects so that they do contribute directly both to hypothesis-making, to formulating the final conclusions, and to what goes on in between . . . . In the complete form of this approach, not only will the subject be fully fledged co-researcher, but the researcher will also be co-subject, participating fully in the action and experience to be researched. (Heron, 1981: 19–20)

The relationships between all actors in the process of practice must be such as to generate together critical thinking, reflection and dialogue.

Ahmed advocates full community involvement in reviews of the delivery of social services to black people (Ahmed, 1989). Reciprocal arrangements within such reviews should go beyond the full dissemination of results in appropriate languages. They should include measures to strengthen the ability of people to participate, such as payment, the provision of technical assistance to the community, and training. Ahmed suggests that these can help to neutralise the charges of exploitation, racism and elitism – all terms which can function as opposites of reciprocity. The use of indigenous interviewers, as well as being more effective, can also have some potential for contributing something to the community and possibly empowering some of its residents (Ahmed, 1989: 27–8). A survey of elders is recalled in which the interviewers themselves, through highlighting the needs they were uncovering, gained training and personal development. In some cases this led to professional employment. The community as a whole gained a slowly improved understanding of barriers to an effective service in those statutory and voluntary agencies which were asked to contribute to the training.

Participating with others in processes of knowledge construction implies rejecting negative labels and seeing people as strong, capable and informative. O'Hagan (1986) gives an example based on her decision fully to involve psychiatric survivors in her study of patients' experiences and the need for a user-run advocacy organisation. The decision to depart from her original, conventional proposal was taken for various reasons, including the fact that 'They had no opportunity within the research structure to think through their experience. Yet most of them were thoughtful people who were capable of it' (O'Hagan, 1986: 18). By seeing the strengths in people, she was able to add many rich and valuable strands to her research and to produce a more significant outcome. To put her perspective into practice and have it taken seriously by the researched, however, she had to give away some of her power. She passed final control over the research proposal and over the editing of write-ups to the survivors' group (O'Hagan, 1986: 24). She was embarrassed to reflect that, despite being a psychiatric survivor herself, the role of conventional researcher placed her in the same controlling relationship over those whose experience she was researching as professionals had over her: 'Like a mental illness worker I probed, selected and extracted and made judgements, without the informed consent or involvement of the interviewee' (O'Hagan, 1986: 23). Her revised and fully participatory approach will be returned to later in this chapter.

As Heron puts it,

> Traditional research on persons is a way of exercising power . . . Research . . . becomes another agent of authoritarian social control. Knowledge and power are all on the side of the researchers and their political masters, and none is on the side of those who provide the data and are subject to its subsequent application . . . the moral principle of respect for persons is most fully honoured when power is shared not only in the application of knowledge about persons, but also in the generation of such knowledge. (Heron, 1981: 34–5)

The pursuit of participatory approaches is fundamentally the pursuit of power sharing. If research-minded practice is not developed as such, the powerful alliance of research and practice brings with it dangers of greater social control.

The commitment to anti-oppressive working must be absolute for the research-minded practitioner. Mies, a feminist researcher, makes a very similar argument to that of Nicolaus (1972) referred to in Chapter 4:

> Research, which has so far been largely an instrument of dominance and legitimation of power elites, must be brought to serve the interests of dominated, exploited and oppressed groups . . . . Women scholars, committed to the cause of women's liberation, cannot have an objective interest in a 'view from above'. This would mean that they would consent to their own oppression as women, because the man–woman relationship represents one of the oldest examples of the view from above. (Mies, 1983: 123)

In Chapter 2 we reflected on the argument that according credibility to the views of the less powerful will enhance what we know: they have their own perspectives on the world and also will have developed understandings of the behaviour and perspectives of those who oppress them (Nielsen, 1990). Second, having regard for people in the research process will lead to their becoming less suspicious of the whole process (Mies, 1983: 123 reminds us that distrust is further augmented by social class difference). Third, those with the experience know which questions matter and can consequently help to ask and answer them. A study of day care needs of women returning to work (Mullender, 1990) includes a commitment to avoiding obtaining only the views of employers and public officials. The voice of the women themselves is arguably the most crucial. They will help to set the terms of the project, in language which makes sense to them and reflects their own experience and understanding (Pease, 1990).

Working with young people leaving care, Stein and Carey (1986) made an explicit decision not to seek any external validation of the views of the young people they were interviewing about their experiences. There was no wish to provide any explanations which competed with those of the young people themselves. This is a clear statement of values and reflects the 'view from below'. In a review of the published study, however, Fruin (1987) regrets the decision not to incorporate 'triangulation' (different ways of collecting data on the same issue to ensure more reliable results). In his view, this 'would have had the merit of adding others' perspectives on the same sequences of events and could thereby have strengthened the study's conclusions and prescriptions for change' (Fruin, 1987: 556). This is a matter of opinion and that opinion rests on values. Stein and Carey's aim was to give a voice to users, as a matter of principle, and this was achieved. O'Hagan, on the other hand, felt she made progress when she moved from interviewing only psychiatric survivors to including families and professionals and – most importantly in the development of her research process – having them all come together to discuss the issues involved: 'the picture takes on a new form and a fuller meaning. Knowledge grows' (O'Hagan, 1986: 19).

Fruin's comments that, as recognised by the authors, there were no black care-leavers in their sample and no-one facing the additional rigours of life in a large city carry more weight (Fruin, 1987). We might expect black and inner city young people to face special problems and their knowledge of these is crucial to planning better services.

Language itself is data and may be subjected to close analysis. We can learn much about the ways people act and react from the way they conceptualise their own actions and contexts. Sims (1981) gives an interesting account of just such a process. He studied the subject of problem construction by listening to health service professionals talking about their own team's difficulties – and slipped into action research when he began feeding back his observations.

Purposes

The first question in undertaking participatory or indeed any research should always be 'What is the purpose of the research?' So the research-minded practitioner will constantly be asking the question 'What is the purpose of this practice?'

Clear reasons for practising must underpin decisions as to what kind of data is needed and how best to obtain it. In Chapter 3 we argued that, in practice as in research, where values are to the fore, the question 'why?' must assume equal importance with the questions 'what?' and 'how?' In research we cannot jump from deciding what is to be studied to the technical how questions. We cannot select the tools for the job without first considering why we are asking the questions in the first place and what we hope to find out. Neither can we decide on what services are to be delivered, in what ways and by whom, without considering – why these services?

There are other questions, too, which we will also find it instructive to ask. Different interest groups represented in practice may all favour different forms of data. Funding agencies may prefer to see formalised statistics being gathered; managers may be seeking to find out what forms of intervention are effective; service users may want to expose an unacceptable philosophy underlying current service delivery. A further question is whether the work of the research-minded practitioner leaves service users stronger than before. This forms a constant theme throughout this chapter. All the questions here require careful reflection before an appropriate range of data collection techniques is selected. All can affect what we need to know and how we can get to know it.

There is a tendency to equate data gathering with questionnaires, yet there is a great deal more to the process than this. Data are frequently gathered without thought being given to the processes employed. It is important not to jump in without closely considering which tools are best for which purposes. All the major data-gathering techniques are well explained in a standard way by Shipman (1988) and in a participative way by Wadsworth (1984) and Feuerstein (1986). Their combined use in an educational setting is well documented by Burgess (1984).

The three classic approaches to collecting data – observation, asking questions (by interview or questionnaire) and analysing documentary sources – are designed to do different jobs. The following example describes two of them being combined to collect detailed consumer feedback as well as the researcher's own impressions of consumer satisfaction:

> The users' views were obtained in a variety of ways. First, through direct observation of Drop-in life over a period of four months; second, through informal conversations with users individually and in groups; third, through tape-recorded, semi-structured interviews in the users' own homes. The latter were designed to gather material about the users' families, how they spent their time, which agencies and other networks they contacted for help, how they came to use the Drop-in and their views on how it had satisfied their needs. (Cigno, 1988: 365)

Masses of information will have been gathered in this study, some factual but most of it more subjective – and not a questionnaire in sight.

In the above example it is clear that learning about personal experience of the drop-in facility was an important goal of the study and that techniques of data collection were selected accordingly. O'Hagan's monograph (1986) on her personal journey from a traditional to a more unconventional and participatory approach is a valuable reflection on researching personal experience, both that of users and of the researcher. Traditional research tends to miss the personal stories, the narrative histories and subjective meanings which lie behind day-to-day events. Participatory and feminist research values them more highly. Such work can give a voice to previously silenced and disempowered service users if the research-minded practitioner can find the methods and develop the right orientation for this to happen.

Assessments in practice are based on the same mixture of radically different kinds of information and impressions as research: whether gleaned from observing someone in their own home, listening to their personal account of what has happened to them, liaising with others who know them, or reading their case file. Dean and Fenby discuss how social work students can be encouraged to consider whether they are in pursuit primarily of facts or the meanings those facts carry for service users. Participants in a child abuse case may recount different versions of events either because they are departing from the truth or because they see the world differently. The student, argue Dean and Fenby, needs an awareness of varying epistemological positions, or world views, in order to balance his or her concerns with historical and with narrative truth. They conclude that history taking and assessment can be taught in many different ways, beginning from students examining their past practice and deciding whether they veer towards empirical or existential ways of knowing (Dean and Fenby, 1989).

A further example encompasses most of the techniques likely to be used by social work researchers: observation, questionnaires, interviews and the use of documentation. In studying a particular model of social action groupwork, the researcher attended group meetings, interviewed workers and members, and worked in one of the groups herself as a participant observer. She gathered additional data from published accounts of the groups concerned, from the groups' own records, from publicity materials and newsletters they had produced, and from their amassed 'memorabilia' which included photographs, letters, drawings and jottings.

Shipman (1988) reminds us that interrogating documents is essentially the same process as asking questions in an interview: what was the author's perspective or bias, their motivation for writing, and their degree of proximity to the actual events described? Wadsworth (1984) cautions similarly that in examining agency documents we may be encountering official views of reality or the vested interests of management. Taking evidence from ordinary people or from basic grade workers might produce quite different accounts. Documentation may be pre-existing (for example, public or agency records, case files, minutes of staff or committee meetings, memoranda and circulars, job descriptions) or produced for the purposes of the research (for example, personal accounts, drink diaries, activity sheets covering a typical day, journals; see O'Hagan 1986). Given that social workers often have ready access to audio-visual equipment, they may also consider generating data through taping a meeting, or series of meetings, or other activities, for later analysis of interactions. Here the people concerned would need to be fully involved in discussing ethics and consents in advance and in controlling the recording process. Photographs, audio and video tapes may also provide important evidence about a style of social work intervention and its use in practice. Pattern analysis of verbal interaction between worker and user, or analysis at the non-verbal level, can help to indicate whether or not the practitioner is on the right wavelength and demonstrating empathy – though both concepts would be hard to define.

Shipman also mentions the use of unobtrusive measures, that is evidence which people leave lying all around them in the course of daily life. An example which would be very relevant in a study of alcohol abuse is counting empty bottles in the dustbin (Shipman, 1988: 114). Another example might be observing the degree of visible stimulation in a study of the quality of life in a residential setting. Such data are valuable as additional information where triangulation, the use of more than one technique and source, is desirable. There is no limitation on data-gathering techniques, particularly where we call on the imaginations of all participants.

Communication

Practitioners, perhaps more than researchers, already have so many of the necessary skills and the willingness to engage with others as 'people first' (to borrow a phrase from a field of learning difficulties), rather than as the 'subjects' or 'objects' of research. It is far easier to encourage someone to speak openly and honestly, and far easier really to hear what they are saying, if they are accorded

respect and treated as people with abilities with something important to offer.

A graphic example is provided by a piece of research to advise on
the employment and training-related needs of people with learning
difficulties. The decision had been taken to establish a new project
but, rather than replicate ideas which had not proved tremendously
successful in the past, it was agreed that there should be a fresh
analysis of the issues, followed by a feasibility study. The researcher,
strongly committed to a participatory style, both in practice and
research, felt that the work should directly involve people with
learning difficulties or risk being both patronising and inappropriate. A user-led, self-advocacy project entered into a partnership
with the researcher. Communication skills, with appropriate values,
emphasised the strengths in people, rejected negative labels and
believed that people acting together could be powerful, and that all
work should be anti-oppressive. It took two meetings and the best
part of a day to write and word process the letter accepting the
commission to launch the work. But the letter truly represented the
views of all concerned and was produced by the people with
learning difficulties themselves. Their involvement should mean
that the end result of the work is more relevant and includes: the
identification of a core group of people to establish a self-advocacy
project in the researched area; a sample user response to the new
proposals; the development of action packages, including models of
communication, support and information sharing; and a series of
skills input workshops. Without open communication and challenging values, there might have been only another dusty report on a
shelf.

Social work has both the commitment and the ability to communicate with people who are relatively powerless. All participatory
researchers hold this as an aim, but practitioners should be well
equipped to achieve it. Non-verbal aspects of communication may
be important here. For example, reading the signs that a young
person who has been in trouble with the law is still feeling hesitant
about confiding in someone apparently 'in authority' may clarify
for the practitioner that the proposed young people's social action
project should be jointly designed and managed before expecting
commitment to it. Likewise, the patience to talk to a disabled
person who is an expert on the issues of independent living, but
whose speech may be slow and indistinct, would be taken for
granted by most social workers and could make a tremendous
contribution to understandings and to informed practice.

The commitment to anti-oppressive working also means that inequalities in interpersonal communication be addressed. Spender (1980), for example, shows how men dominate conversations and interrupt more often than women. Interpreters must be employed in racially mixed communities. Vocabularies (argot) which develop among sub-cultural groupings, such as prisoners or even young people in care, need to be acknowledged. The research-minded practitioner also needs to be open to the kind of communication which may arise from the experience of oppression itself and not try to sanitise or translate this into safer or more familiar expressions. Anger is allowable.

This morning's session on mental health research was a discussion by several researchers who seemed squarely and securely fenced in by convention . . . The oppressed are free to know differently. While their oppressors need to keep their dominant knowledge to survive as oppressors, the oppressed need to create a new knowledge to stop their oppression. This is essential for self-determination. (O'Hagan, 1986: 16–17)

There are significant issues involved in the internal communication styles of groups. In studies of formal groups and organisations, O'Hagan (1986) shows how patterns of communication adopted internally often owe more to people's desire to maintain their position in the pecking order than to their efforts to clarify or achieve tasks. Thus, in a discussion between mental health policy makers and professionals, the former group slipped into defending and the latter into attacking. Rather than looking at each other's point of view, they were a million miles from joining to explore what philosophy and quality of service users would like to see or how these could most effectively be achieved. O'Hagan concludes that 'the hierarchical structuring of knowledge and power . . . distorts the communication experience; isolates the people on different levels from one another and invalidates the experiences of those on the lower levels' (O'Hagan, 1986: 27). This will have a marked impact on the research-minded practitioner who attempts to study, intervene in, or communicate with the organisation at any or all levels and who wishes to see services become less oppressive.

O'Hagan (1986) favours a research style which establishes lines of communication not only backwards and forwards, between researcher and researched, but in all directions, including between the different groups under study. She advocates bringing everyone together in sub-groups and in the total group to exchange ideas and see what new insights can be derived. This is not a naive attempt to smooth out all discord. She gives one example (O'Hagan, 1986: 13) where the process of communication led the positions of users and relatives to become polarised on the topics of self-advocacy and compulsory committal. This division of views was crucial and needed to be revealed in the research, just as it would need to be in practice.

Roles

Research-minded practitioners play the role not of directors but of facilitators of a critical, reflective process. Rather than imposing their own aims or direction, they draw out strengths in those formally excluded from decision making and help them determine what they want the practice to achieve. They regard service users as having expertise and ideas. Their own key contribution is the privilege of time to think, the responsibility to involve others creatively in this process and the skill to encourage people to discover what they are capable of achieving.

The facilitator's role allows scope for working with the pre-existing leadership structure in a natural group without undermining it or challenging it in a damaging way. There may be times when people may have to consider whether to accept what the practitioner has to offer, particularly if they have had previously bad experiences of professionals. Once engaged in a joint piece of work, one of the roles of the practitioner will be to encourage those involved to speak out about their lives and the problems which confront them. This provides a means of altering agendas towards their concerns rather than those of the service delivery agency.

This way of working can feel very time-consuming and frustrating. Developments would often be quicker and more predictable if the professional, be they researcher or practitioner, went ahead and took decisions. The refusal to be directive can be difficult for all parties, but the process is nonetheless necessary if service users are to take responsibility for decisions and outcomes. Good practice and good research have the same values and can become the same process. There is no methodological reason why every piece of intervention should not also become a piece of research. Interpretive and feminist research makes the inclusion of personal experience acceptable, provided it is recorded and analysed with the same degree of rigour as any other form of information. In feminist research, personal experience of both the researched and the researcher are fundamental. O'Hagan remarks: 'After several interviews I realised that I had thought through my experience as a psychiatric survivor more than most of the interviewees. It seemed a waste not to include it in the research data' (O'Hagan, 1986: 18). Reinharz, from a feminist perspective, describes the process of self-critical reflection:

> the researcher investigates his/her own previous experiences, intentions, hopes, prejudices to try to understand what s/he is bringing to the study . . . . S/he also keeps a personal diary throughout the research process, keeping close touch with changing attitudes . . . . The record of the researcher's feelings and ideas is also data, a clue to the nature of the social environment being studied . . . . Many of one's predispositions, when known, can be questions put to the persons one is studying – they need not be discarded. They are only 'biases' if they are not acknowledged or explored, as is almost always the case in positivist research. (Reinharz, 1983: 175–6)

Practitioners, when they have undertaken research, have often found it difficult to adopt the role of the detached researcher. Sainsbury and his colleagues stepped out of the research role on such urgent occasions as the discovery of live wires sticking out of a wall or an imminent eviction. But these are seen as aberrations: 'In the vast majority of cases, however, we consider that we remained detached interviewers' (Sainsbury *et al.*, 1982: 9). These researchers had almost entirely sloughed their social work skins: 'Both research-interviewers had been practising social workers and were occasionally considerably tempted to adopt this role' (Sainsbury *et al.*, 1982: 9).

We are writing for a readership still wearing the identity of a practitioner. In any case, the urge to intervene goes deeper than a paid job or a need to interfere. It is also related to the underpinning purposes and values of the piece of work. The principles of action research can provide a solution here, in that action is combined with evaluation. The former does not have to wait until the latter has duly weighed its deliberations and reported to its commissioning sponsors. This is more in keeping with the ethics of social work. We should be unaccustomed to passing by on the other side and, whilst medical research may demand that some patients go untreated whilst acting as the controls in tests of new drugs, action research, by combining the 'complexity of real experience' with 'striving for concrete improvement' (McTaggart, 1982: 6), provides a way round this in our profession. In research-minded practice, participants become active partners in the process of critical enquiry:

the distinction between researcher and researched is broken down. The only difference between my roles and the roles of the other participants is that I will be also the coordinator and compiler. These roles could also be shared. (O'Hagan, 1986: 18)

O'Hagan introduced an 'inverted hierarchy' into her research whereby the psychiatric survivors had more roles than the other researched groups and the final say in decision making, including that over the research proposal and any associated publications.

Skills

Adopting the values we have outlined in Chapter 3 is not easy. The chief skill is involving people fully in the process. In action research, for example, the major impact of change is sought through such ongoing involvement and not at the much later stage of disseminating someone else's research findings (Kemmis 1984: 27). People are directly involved at the time when the issue to be studied is real and its dilemmas are acute, not months later when the situation may already have eased or various solutions have been tried with varying and by now untestable degrees of success.

Further skills required in data collection include those of listening, observing, recording, clarifying and interpreting. They must always be applied in a value-informed way which implies working jointly with the people involved in the process. Recording, for example, is not a private matter of the practitioner or researcher keeping notes and files on the information gathered. The process and style of recording, and the location of responsibility for carrying it out, need to be arrived at in a shared way. Information needs to be accessible to all the participants, and all relevant people need to understand the information-retrieval system and framework for analysis. It may be agreed that it is acceptable for the research-minded practitioner to keep his or her own log of tasks undertaken, issues raised and indications for future work. At the same time, some of this material may also be fed in at intervals for a shared review of progress to date on the project. The ethical principles underlying the recording also need to be explored together. In a user-run mental health project, for example, the basic principle of the workers was not to divulge identifying information on users. The outside evaluator was still able to gather information from them, however, by making contact through the workers. As he commented:

> The design of the evaluation has to walk a narrow path between the gathering of reliable information sufficient to permit a valid independent judgement, and the insensitive, intrusive insistence on knowing and recording what one has no business to know. (Meikle, 1988: 1)

At every stage of the data-generation and -collection process, a participatory value base can give rise to enriched understanding. It can also release the potential for action, unimpeded by long delays and assisted by conceptualisation of real relevance to the work in hand. A research approach can be used to demystify both practice and evaluation if admissible knowledge is defined, and measures designed, with the full participation of service users. Where this happens, everyone acquires new skills and learns that the process is not magical but can be varied or repeated in fresh circumstances to generate further information. Decisions are taken jointly about the whole process. This is a more ethical and generally also a more effective way to proceed since:

> concepts like 'discover', 'facts', 'scientific study of a subject' and 'critical investigation' have no value for the weavers of experience. These concepts cannot grasp, let alone validate, all the complex and untidy loose ends of experience. These loose ends must be woven into a patterned web of interconnecting insights and actions. (O'Hagan, 1986: 8)

In the next chapter we will explore how the many strands of the web begin to be brought together through data analysis.

7

Analysing the Data of Practice

Practitioners are engaged in the process of data analysis all of the time. They interpret and assign meaning to all kinds of data from a wide range of sources: what they read, what they see, what they hear, what they are told, what they themselves think and feel. In this chapter we explore ways in which practitioners may become more aware, more explicit and more rigorous about these processes.

Turn to the chapter on data analysis in almost any research methods book and you will find material on the statistical analysis of data: frequency distributions, tables, pie charts, bar diagrams, statistical correlations, calculations of the degrees of probability of the truth of findings (see, for example; Philip, McCulloch and Smith, 1975; Fruin, 1980; Pilcher, 1990).

We have already noted that it can be useful for practice to quantify and statistically analyse data. There may well be times when it seems that the presentation of an argument or analysis of a situation in these terms may be the most meaningful. Decision-making arenas, be they management committees, local authority council meetings, working parties, management groups or public enquiries, often assume models of scientific rationality. Whether this actually reflects the reality of the ways in which decisions are made in these arenas is another story. Nevertheless, it may well be the case that the practitioner decides, in participation with others involved in the particular project, that quantitative and statistical analysis of findings is the most likely way to influence decisions and policy to bring about desired change.

We recall an example in the early 1970s involving community workers and research workers in the London docklands area.

Together with local people, they presented evidence to a public enquiry which included the statistical analysis of data relating to the likely harmful effects on local people of anticipated noise levels with the proposed airport to serve the City of London. The airport has now been built – such is the nature of power and decision making – but it was worth a try. Perhaps more successful outcomes have been achieved in the presentation of statistical data on traffic to support campaigns for the closure of a street to make it safe for children to play.

Reflecting on these examples brings us to two conclusions. First, the quantification and statistical analysis of data should not be rejected out of hand. It may be useful for the purpose. But it is a form of analysis that should be used with a mind to its usefulness. Is it the most meaningful way to understand or present issues? Our concern is that this predominant way of analysing data often alienates practitioners and those with whom they work. It is through this form of analysis that the research process can serve to mystify rather than to enlighten. The fundamental question to be addressed in analysing data is: does this way of understanding and presenting the data shed light on their meaning?

Our second conclusion is about the interests that are served by supposedly scientific rational models of research and decision making. We suggested in Chapter 4 that positivism and the technical rational model impede the pursuit of research for social welfare. Positivist research tends to serve dominant interests in a number of ways. It purports to deal in 'facts' alone; it claims to control variables sufficiently to prove cause and effect; it makes opinions look like facts through translating them into numerical scores; it suggests that 'facts' about the social world are simple concepts with an independent existence of their own; it promotes the view that decisions about, for example, the definition and prevalence of need and the allocation of resources are technical judgements to be made by experts on the basis of social scientific knowledge supposedly not influenced by values and political ideologies (Pease, 1990). Such decisions are political, but are removed from the political agenda and decision-making forum. In other words, research can be used to sanitise decisions, making them appear spuriously scientific. This serves to keep political decisions and value choices out of the hands of ordinary citizens, leaving their interests on trust, in the hands of technical experts.

Numerical scores can be assigned to data that are counted, data that are collected in structured ways (through questionnaires for example) and to more qualitative data. All data can be assigned numerical scores, quantified and analysed statistically. For the research-minded practitioner working in emancipatory ways, there can, though, be dangers in attempting to quantify understandings: allocating numerical 'scores' or values to observations, responses to questionnaires and the like. The effect can be to force subtleties of judgement into predefined categories that are limited by the dimensions anticipated in advance (Campbell, 1979: 50) and the level of understanding of the researcher. All the richness of comprehension and reflection which engaging in dialogue might have contributed is foregone. In this chapter we will explore ways in which this richness can be captured and reflected upon theoretically through participative processes of data analysis.

Analysing data is a matter of capturing the richness of comprehension and reflection. As such, it is not an activity that comes only at the end of the research process when all the data are collected. The process of research, and the practice of the research-minded practitioner, are not like that. As we have said before, research and practice are not linear processes. In leaving data analysis for one of the later chapters of this book, we are adopting the common format of research methods texts. Partly this is only convention. Analysis of data takes place throughout the research process. To emphasise this, we open this chapter by drawing on references to data analysis which we have made in earlier chapters.

In Chapter 4, we drew up the model for the research-minded practitioner. In that chapter we referred to Schon's contrasting descriptions of the positivist, expert practitioner and the reflective practitioner. These descriptions remind us of the reflexive process of data analysis and its centrality throughout the process.

In Chapter 2, we argued that data cannot be taken at their face value. We demonstrated this using Freudian, Marxist and feminist theoretical approaches. Thus we argued that our actions and thoughts are shaped by our unconscious and childhood experiences; by our class position in an ideology-imbued society; and by gender relations and deep-rooted notions of masculinity and femininity in a gender divided society. In the same chapter, we theoretically unpacked the concept of 'race' to show that, despite its having no validity as a biological phenomenon, it is nevertheless powerful in shaping people's experiences and understandings of the world. Race, gender and class are used to divide people and oppress some – they can also be used as forms of resistance, as black people and women have shown.

We repeat this here to stress the importance once again of understanding the social sources of data. Terms used in research texts such as 'raw' and 'pure' data, are misleading in that they imply that data, when first collected, arrive in an uncontaminated form. This is not the case. Data are constructed through social structures, language and processes, the process of the research-minded practitioner. Throughout this book, we have stressed the need to pay attention to the processes through which data are constructed. Our very language, the means we have to describe, and our everyday concepts construct our subjectivities.

The only honest way forward, as well as the most theoretically legitimate and the most illuminating, is for subjective meanings and experiences to be incorporated into the process of getting to know. This includes the subjectivities of both the researcher and the researched. The process of analysing data is one of understanding the ways in which data is constructed and further constructing the data through theoretical categorisation and reflection. Thus data analysis starts at the beginning of the process. Reflecting on the meaning of data is not an activity that comes at the end, but is integral to all the stages of a research-minded process.

There is no such thing as 'pure' research, there are only researchers who choose not to examine the impact of their own views, and those of their sponsors, on the research process. Data are not necessarily what they seem. Their meaning in a society divided by class, race and gender need to be understood. Otherwise, in analysing data, we can be in danger of assuming neutrality in expression – when all we are in fact doing is leaving data impregnated with the dominant values of our society. As we argued in Chapter 4, this process must be carried out in a participative way. Crucial to the process of empowerment is ensuring that people have the opportunity to understand the processes of knowledge production. This relates both to the knowledge of others and that presented to us. It also relates to our own subjectivities.

In Chapter 5, we explored the ways in which research-minded practitioners would explore issues in practice. We suggested that fundamental to their approach would be their awareness, and critical scrutiny, of policy and organisational categorisations of need. In other words, the research-minded practitioner would be alert to interpretations and meanings that have been assigned to data and that are implicit in the application of categories. The opportunity to develop different categories is always possible through practice that is research-minded. We suggested that, in participatory practice, the formulation of problems and issues is a matter of active negotiation of grounded realities. In other words, the issues to be addressed by the research-minded practitioner, working with others, are defined through the process of sharing understandings of social phenomena. The example we gave in Chapter 5 was that concerned with formulating issues around the disproportionate number of black children in care – to be addressed then in rigorous, analytic and questioning practice.

Implicit within the process of engaging with others to generate data, the focus of Chapter 6, is the interconnectedness of data collection and data analysis. In participatory practice, data and their meanings are generated through reciprocal exchange, through dialogue. Observations and interpretations, are shared to establish the ways in which they do, or do not, ring true for everyone. They are contextualised and theorised so that the ways in which views are shaped in an unequal and oppressive society are taken into account. The different perspectives of participants are debated for shared understandings to emerge.

The process of data analysis is to do with detecting patterns in the data. In the course of analysing quantitative data, these patterns will emerge as tables, percentages, bar diagrams, pie charts and tests of significance. The exercise will be different in drawing out patterns in qualitative data. Patterns emerge through the researcher or practitioner becoming familiar with the data and yet, at the same time, being in the position of stranger. 'Making the familiar strange' (Jeffs and Smith, 1990) is crucial to the process of data analysis. It ensures that what might seem obvious questions are put to data whose meaning can so easily be taken for granted. In summary, data analysis is a process of:

● making sense;
● developing meanings;
● identifying patterns and processes;
● addressing multiple and contradictory realities;
● not establishing objective truths but of reaching 'tentative approximations' (Glaser and Strauss, 1967) which are constantly open to further negotiation and revision.

We now return to the model of practice for the practitioner who is research-minded as proposed in Chapter 4 and used in Chapters 5 and 6 to explore the different stages of practice, formulating the issues and engaging with subjects to generate data. In this chapter we reflect on ways in which the practitioner who is research-minded may analyse data in practice in relation to the six aspects of practice identified in our model: values, ethics, purposes, communication, roles and skills. Chapter 3 set out the values for such a practitioner. There is a close relationship between these and the values to be adopted in analysing data. We start by exploring these.

Value base

As suggested above, the process of data analysis may best be seen as one of 'tentative approximations' (Glaser and Strauss, 1967) in which the meaning of data is actively negotiated by participants in the practice, from their different perspectives as managers, practitioners, workers from other agencies or users. Practitioners, adopting the values we espouse in Chapter 3, will be responsible for ensuring that everyone has the opportunity critically to reflect on what is happening in practice. Practitioners who are research-minded have regard for people's everyday understandings of their world. They recognise that the users of social welfare services can contribute to the process of problem formulation and assessment, to decisions about choices of interventions and to definitions of their situations and needs.

The practitioner is central to the process of negotiating meaning or ensuring that participants negotiate together. If the ways in which we know the world (or understand what is happening to us) are influenced, structured and constrained by our place within it, then the research-minded practitioner must be aware of this in the process of negotiating what the data mean to each participant. From this perspective, then, in the data analysis process, practitioners are involved in actively co-producing rather than individually discovering the meaning of their data. Their own assumptions, the assumptions of others and the practice process itself must become parts of an analysis which explicitly addresses the complex nature of multiple realities and different 'truths'.

Sometimes it may be the case that different views are recorded or different truths are presented. Understanding will be enriched by taking account of different ways in which others perceive situations and theoretically analysing the sources and implications of these differences. However, practitioners differ from researchers in that they will often be in the situation where they have to judge between competing views and make decisions in the face of inadequate information. After all, they are accorded the professional responsibility so to do.

Researchers have adopted a number of different positions in relation to the vexed issue of how to judge whose view is closest to reality, having accepted that there is no one 'truth', no essential reality. Becker's position is this: he starts by acknowledging that, in analysing data, there is no one truth, no neutral, value-free position. And so, 'the question is not whether we should take sides, since we inevitably will, but rather whose side are we on' (Becker, 1970: 99). He then reflects on the sympathy he feels, and is accused of, for those he studies (in the field of deviancy) and asks the questions:

Will the research, we wonder be distorted by that sympathy? Will it be of use in the construction of scientific theory or in the application of scientific knowledge to the practical problems of society? Or will the bias introduced by taking sides spoil it for those uses? (Becker, 1970: 100)

These are important and relevant questions for the practitioner. Will my sympathy for those with whom I work (colleagues and clients) distort my judgements of the truth?

In reflecting on the meaning of the accusation of bias, by self or others, Becker reveals that this usually occurs when, through research, credence has been given to the views of the 'underdog', the drug addicts within the system of criminal justice, the pupils in the school, the patients in the hospital (Becker, 1970):

We provoke the charge when we assume, for the purposes of our research, that subordinates have as much right to be heard as superordinates, that they are as likely to be telling the truth as they see it as superordinates, that what they say about the institution has a right to be investigated and have its truth or falsity established, even though responsible officials assure us that it is unnecessary because the charges are false. (Becker, 1970: 102–3)

These are important words for the practitioner who is research-minded. How many injustices have remained unseen because attempts to make them visible have been made by those deemed not to be credible, such as children in children's homes, lower-grade workers in social service and hospital bureaucracies? Becker coins the term 'hierarchy of credibility' to make the point that those at the top are assumed to have a fuller picture of reality than people on the lower rungs, whose views are bound to be partial only. Becker relates this to organisations and also to classes and suggests that accusations of bias are made when the researcher does not accept this hierarchy of credibility – when the established and accepted way of understanding of situations is challenged (Becker, 1970). The accusation is seldom made the other way round since most people in a subordinate position are not organised to make the accusation of bias of the researcher who 'favors officialdom' (Becker, 1970: 105). In response to the reply that the researcher should present all views – those of the subordinates but also those of the superordinates – Becker is clear about who does not tell the truth:

> Because they are responsible in this way, officials usually have to lie. That is a gross way of putting it, but not inaccurate. Officials must lie because things are seldom as they ought to be. For a variety of reasons, well-known to sociologists, institutions are refractory. They do not perform as society would like them to. Hospitals do not cure people; prisons do not rehabilitate prisoners; schools do not educate students. Since they are supposed to, officials develop ways both of denying the failure of the institution to perform as it should and explaining those failures which cannot be hidden. An account of an institution's operation from the point of view of subordinates therefore casts doubt on the official line and may possibly expose it as a lie. (Becker, 1970: 104–105)

In Chapter 2 and in Chapter 6, we referred to the feminist standpoint epistemological position which develops this point in relation to gender and race. Feminist standpoint theorists accord validity to the perspectives of women and black people on the grounds that these people not only understand their own experiences but also learn to understand the experiences of those who dominate them.

Ethics

In a research-minded way, we can be prepared to disrupt 'hierarchies of credibility'. But this leaves us with two problems. The first is that hierarchies are infinite. We are not just talking about

Directors of Social Services and workers, or workers and users: we are also talking about husbands and wives, parents and children, adolescents and young children, white kids and black kids. The second is that to suggest that absolute truth rests with the 'underdog' is to deny what we learnt in Chapter 2 about the ways in which subjectivities are shaped and constructed through language, social processes and structures. As there is no objective reality, so there is also no essential subject. When we have responsibilities to act in what are being revealed by subordinates as abusive situations, how do we judge the truth?

There is no answer. However, ethical practice on the part of the practitioner who is research-minded would involve:

● being as well informed as possible with information systematically and rigorously acquired;
● having regard for the views of those who, in our society, are all too often accorded so little credibility;
● being rigorous in taking into account as many views as possible from those who may have a perspective on the situation;
● understanding the ways in which some people are more articulate than others and that views are constructed through social structures, processes and experiences, and sharing these understandings with those involved;
● being theoretically informed, able to call on a range of theories that would possibly contribute understandings to the situation;
● being alert to the tendency to choose from theories in an eclectic way, drawing only from those aspects that support your own beliefs;
● being alert to the tendency to practise routinely, calling on the favourite theories of the time and intervening in familiar ways;
● reaching judgement through reason and argument; and
● being publicly accountable for the judgement and the processes that have been pursued in reaching it.

Purposes

Data have to be analysed for them to make sense. The process of analysis is one of interpreting data, assigning meaning to them, making sense of them. In this chapter and throughout this book we have stressed the importance of the practitioner engaging with others in a participative way to negotiate meanings. The process of analysis should be visible and explicit. It should be open for others to participate in and be available for scrutiny, interrogation and change. In the section below on communication we will explore these processes of negotiatión further. Here we focus on the purpose of analysing data rigorously and systematically.

Hammersley and Atkinson suggest that the purpose of analysing data is one of reflexivity. Their experience is in undertaking qualitative research in school classrooms (Hammersley and Atkinson, 1983). For us the similarity between the researcher's reflexive approach and that of the reflective practitioner (Schon, 1983) is important. The process of reflexivity recognises that researchers, or practitioners who are research-minded, are part of the social world which they are seeking to understand.

Two things follow. First: 'we must work with what knowledge we have, whilst recognising that it may be erroneous and subjecting it to systematic inquiry where doubt seems justified' (Hammersley and Atkinson, 1983: 15). Most data that the practitioner reflects upon remain unrecorded. In interpreting the world, drawing conclusions and making inferences, practitioners rely a great deal on memory. The problem is that memory is selective and we select in ways that fit data to our preconceived ideas, what we expect to find, our cherished beliefs, common sense. In analysing data, it is important to try to take account of as many data as possible and to be particularly attentive to those data which may confuse us, surprise us or make us less certain. In everyday life, it is these data that are often overlooked and forgotten. Our assumptions, our beliefs, our hunches, what we have always thought, common sense, also constitute data and must also be subject to rigorous inquiry and analysis. We must always be on the look out for data that may contradict what we would have thought would be the situation, what we have always known.

The second thing which follows from recognising our own place in the situation we are trying to understand is to realise that 'how people respond to the presence of the researcher may be as informative as how they react to other situations' (Hammersley and Atkinson, 1983: 15). Positivist researchers have regarded this as unwanted interference of the researcher and treated the researcher as a variable to be controlled. Qualitative researchers recognise, as practitioners do, that their relationships with those with whom they generate data are important. Practitioners have much to learn from reflecting on the way people react to them.

Reflexivity in practice (Hammersley and Atkinson, 1983) is very much a process of theorising in action (Schon, 1983). It involves:

● deriving hypotheses (tentative interpretations) from our existing knowledge to describe and explain what we read, see and hear and engaging in a process continually to test out the validity of these interpretations against further data;
● reflecting on the products of our participation in generating data about the situation we are seeking to understand, observing our own activities 'from the outside', at least in anticipation or retrospect (see Hammersley and Atkinson, 1983: 17).

Communication

We have stressed ways in which analysis of data takes place throughout practice. It takes the form of interrelating theories with data. Prior knowledge, hunches, guesses and assumptions guide the practitioner in collecting data. Data are then reflected upon, ideas are changed, and further data collected. Thus, theory building and data collection are dialectically linked (Hammersley and Atkinson, 1983: 174).

The reader may wish to refer back to Chapter 2 in which we explored Marxist and feminist epistemologies. Marxists have stressed the dialectical relationship people have with the social world and developed the methodology of praxis: engaging in the world, reflecting upon it, changing the world through continued engagement. Feminists stress the personal as political and the grounding of theorising in subjective experiences. They have developed methodologies of intersubjectivity between women as ways of generating and analysing data. We learn from these epistemological approaches that, for emancipatory practice, the dialectical relationship between theory and data demands a dialogue between all those involved.

Participating with others in exploring theories, assumptions and hypotheses, and continually testing these out and refining them in the light of a wide variety of data from different sources, is fundamental. It is ethical and the only way to ensure validity. Empowerment implies that the process of data analysis will be used to accord everyone the right to know. Everyone's understandings are taken into account and the validity of different subjective understandings is acknowledged. If we listen carefully to what others have to say, to their accounts of their experiences, these will typically contain meanings which have not hitherto been taken into account. This is not to say that each individual subjective account is sovereign. Subjectivities need to be explored to be understood – through processes that are open and publicly accountable.

Merely to appeal to practitioners to be open about interpretations they make of people's experiences denies the complexity of communication, particularly in stressful situations. What is said may not necessarily be the same as what is heard or what is understood; or what is wanting to be heard and understood. Data analysis has actively to take this into account. Practitioners must be sensitive in conveying bad news and be aware that decisions about openness in communication rest not only with them as conveyors of information but also with those expected to be on the receiving end. In communicating meanings, we must be open to a range of different and conflicting interpretations of what ostensibly seems to be the same situation.

Practitioners often cope with telling bad news by routinising the process. While this may be one way of handling volatile and painful situations, people can often cope with a higher degree of explanation, involvement, clarification and reciprocity. Respect for people in these situations is the hallmark of good practice.

Roles

The practitioner who is research-minded plays many roles in relation to data analysis, typically those of educator, enabler and facilitator. These will involve practitioners in developing their abilities to make sense of data and sharing these abilities with others – users, colleagues, managers and workers from other agencies.

Practitioners will also be concerned to enable users to obtain information that is relevant to them. This may be information that is held confidentially in departmental papers; it may be information that rests implicitly in the assumptions of people in positions to make decisions that affect the lives of users. One way of achieving this might be to empower service users to seek more information for themselves. Another means might be to attempt to influence managers, colleagues and workers in other agencies to change the ways in which information is given or withheld.

The educative, enabling and facilitative roles in data analysis will involve practitioners in education and conscientisation programmes:

> The use of the word 'conscientization' stresses the rejection of blind ideological indoctrination, of bureaucratic dogmatism and also of often inefficient spontaneous actions. It points at the development of the creativity of the oppressed in their process of acquiring power to transform structures and mentalities. (IN-ODEP, 1981)

Such programmes would be concerned with developing ways to understand the sources and structural dynamics of everyday understandings. They would open up for people the possibilities for alternative meanings and, thus, possible alternative ways of dealing with private troubles and public ills.

Skills

Hammersley and Atkinson provide us with an example of testing out hypotheses, or theorising in action, recognisable to all of us. This example illustrates the skill involved in being reflexive, or theorising in action:

> Thus, for example, if we know something about school classrooms we can guess that a pupil raising his or her hand may be indicating that he or she is offering to answer a teacher's question, volunteering to do some chore, or owning up to some misdemeanour. To find out which of these applies, or whether some other description is more appropriate, we have to investigate the context in which the action occurs; that is, we have to generate possible meanings from the culture for surrounding or other apparently relevant actions. Having done that, we must then compare the possible meanings for each action and decide which form the most plausible underlying pattern. Thus, to take a simple example, if the teacher has just asked a question, we might conclude that the pupil is offering to provide the answer. If, however, the teacher chooses someone else to answer who successfully provides an answer and yet the original pupil keeps

his or her hand up, we might suspect that the original intention had not been to answer the question but that he or she has something else to say. However, it may be that the pupil is dreaming and has not realised the question has been answered, or it may be that he or she thinks the answer provided was incorrect or has something to add to it. These alternative hypotheses can, of course, be tested by further observations and perhaps also by asking the pupil involved. (Hammersley and Atkinson, 1983: 16)

There are a number of lessons that may be drawn from this example:

● we call upon our existing knowledge to understand what we see;
● our immediate understandings may not be correct – we quickly come to conclusions about situations with which we have become familiar. We must not jump to these conclusions. They may be mistaken;
● we need to know something of the context to understand the behaviour of individuals;
● we must continually try to put our interpretations to the test by seeking more data.

And we must be prepared to put the interpretations of others – managers, colleagues, workers in other agencies and users – to the test. Emancipatory practice does not mean going along with what we are expected to think, how we are expected to understand the world, what line we are expected to adopt. Neither does it mean regarding the views of the 'underdog' as sovereign. Nor does it mean being sentimental about their views. As Becker warns:

We can, for a start, try to avoid sentimentality. We are senti-mental when we refuse, for whatever reason, to investigate some matter that should properly be regarded as problematic. We are sentimental, especially, when our reason is that we would prefer not to know what is going on, if to know would be to violate some sympathy whose existence we may not even be aware of. Whatever side we are on, we must use our techniques impartially enough that a belief to which we are especially sympathetic could be proved untrue. We must always inspect our work carefully enough to know whether our techniques and theories are open enough to allow that possibility. (Becker, 1967: 110)

In the next chapter we consider ways in which practitioners who are research-minded may build in processes of evaluation. Evaluation, too, requires that judgements be made about different perspectives on the effectiveness of a project or piece of work. It also means not being sentimental about existing practices and services. They may no longer be effective.

8

The Practitioner–Evaluator

Unlike aspects of practice covered in preceding chapters – problem formulation, engagement with subjects, analysis – evaluation is invariably informed by research methodologies. Research and evaluation go together. In this chapter we develop a model which moves responsibility for evaluation from the external 'expert' or the top-down manager to the practitioner and her team.

The dominant model of evaluation

The history of evaluation in social work in the UK has been short and episodic. The first major published attempt to evaluate the effectiveness of social work was the quasi-experimental study of social work with the elderly, *Helping the Aged* (Goldberg, 1970). Elderly people referred to a local authority welfare department were assigned to one of two groups, a control group and an experimental one. The evaluation study compared the outcomes of social work undertaken by well-qualified social workers (with the experimental group) with those of untrained welfare workers (the control group). The study found that there was little difference in outcome. Whether elderly people lived longer or whether they maintained or enhanced their social relationships with others, for example, did not appear to be related to their having the attention of a well qualified social worker or not. These findings, which questioned the effectiveness of professional social work and social work education, mirrored the findings of similarly designed evaluation studies undertaken in the United States (Meyer *et al.*, 1965; Reid and Shyne, 1969). Although *Helping the Aged* and similar studies were important and significant in introducing evaluation to UK social work, these evaluation models have hardly impinged on either the practices of social workers or the organisations which employ or fund them. Social workers have tended to turn their backs on evaluation, as they have done with research. A major reason for this is the epistemological base of this dominant mode of evaluation. This approach to evaluation is positivist in design and execution. Similarly it assumes technical and rational forms of both social work and policy decision making. This is illustrated by reflecting upon key features of this dominant model:

● Evaluation is undertaken by an outside 'objective' expert: the practitioner's only involvement is as provider of data and perhaps reader of the published work.

● It is assumed that the evaluator will observe but not influence practice. This raises ethical questions about whether an evaluator, in striving for objectivity, should remain silent when comment or feedback may lead to an improved service for the user. For evaluators to store up their thinking until the end also limits the developmental potential of evaluation.

● The quasi-experimental design not only raises ethical issues about the manipulation of service users, but also assumes that the lives of users, with an infinite number of intervening variables, can indeed be controlled for the purposes of the evaluation.

● Even when quasi-experimental designs are not adopted (Fisher *et al.*, 1986), the emphasis in other designs on input, outcomes and criteria for measurement tries to be too tidy about complex processes. For example, objectives and criteria will emerge, change, become fine-tuned or be rejected, during the process of practice. The dominant evaluation model can be too static and constraining. As such it can fail to capture the dynamic nature of practice and can miss the opportunity to contribute to the creativity of practice. Practice is not neat and tidy.

● The language and method of the research model mystifies evaluation. In its demands on practitioner time, research resources and the very practice itself having to fit in with it, it is not amenable to being built into practice processes.

● Practice is decontextualised: separated for evaluation from its social, political and economic context. Evaluation then produces limited knowledge of the real situation of practice.

● Assumptions are made that policy as well as practice is neat and tidy, technical and rational. It is assumed that 'better decisions depend on better information' (Seebohm, 1968) and that decisions are made on the basis of expertise.

● Evaluation from the outside separates the knowers from the doers, theory from practice. Practitioners experience the model as alienating and irrelevant to the complexity and contradictions of their work.

As a response to these concerns, two alternative approaches to evaluation have emerged: the action–research model and the consumer studies model.

Emerging responses: the action–research model

Two early examples of action–research are the educational priority area programme (Halsey, 1972) and the National Community Development Project (CDP) (National Community Development Project, 1973). Action–research seeks to combine social research with social action. This is not without its problems. As described in Chapter 1, there were fierce debates within the CDP as to the appropriate relationship between action and research. Some argued for the policy science model which had similarities with the dominant evaluation model. Others argued for research as critical ongoing reflection of practice in context. Marris and Rein present just the same debates about the research component of the American War on Poverty:

> Social action is more an endless exploration than the search for solutions to specific problems. We know where we start from, and in what direction we are heading, but we cannot know where we will end up. In the face of ignorance, then, the most rational decisions are those which leave open the greatest range of future choice. And this freedom depends upon a refusal to commit oneself irrevocably to ends as well as means, since they react upon each other in a continual redefinition of the nature of the situation. (Marris and Rein, 1967: 204)

Thus, Marris and Rein replace explicit supposed (or imposed) clarity with ignorance, certainty of purpose with tentative exploratory action. The action–research model recognises that practice is 'tentative, non-committal and adaptive' (Marris and Rein, 1967: 205).

The model of action–research in evaluation, sometimes known as illuminative, responsive or holistic, has developed significantly almost to become a paradigm competing with the dominant model (Parlett and Hamilton, 1976). It recognises that practice is complex and ever-changing and that evaluation of practice will and should influence it in an ongoing way. Thus the evaluator in action–research does not endeavour to remain outside practice and does not seek to objectify it. Terms such as 'independent', 'impartial' and 'critical' replace 'detached', 'objective' and 'neutral' to describe the stance of the evaluator.

In some CDPs, the model of action–research was taken even further. Rather than making distinctions between action and research, all workers developed roles as action-researchers. In this model 'the use of research in facilitating social change at all levels was seen as paramount' (Chapman and Green, 1990: 6). This model of action–research does not superimpose research on action, nor action on research. The approaches and methods of the researcher – explicit theorising, conceptualisation, problem formulation, rigour in data collection and analysis – are built into practice. Thus action–research demands that practice and research change, each taking account of and being informed by the other.

Emerging responses: the client's view

The Client Speaks, published in 1970, is as significant as *Helping the Aged* in the history of evaluation in social work (Mayer and Timms, 1970). It was the first study of the effectiveness of social work in the UK to have sought the consumer view. Given that market research is the major form of social research in the Western world, it is indeed quite extraordinary that it was not until the early 1970s that the views of consumers were thought to have some possible relevance.

Mayer and Timms suggest a number of reasons why consumers of social work had not previously been asked for their opinions:

● Social work had, since the 1920s, been heavily influenced by psychoanalysis which 'encouraged practitioners to discount or explain away views the client might express' (Mayer and Timms, 1970: 14).

● Concern for professional status combined with weaknesses in the social work knowledge base had the effect of social workers defending their territory and claiming that only they knew what was right for the client,

● The individualisation of much of social work developed it as a private activity, with the social worker assuming ownership of the client,

● Positivism of social work research, with its emphasis on quantitative and experimental methods, had militated against the conduct of exploratory studies of a qualitative nature such that attention has been drawn away from seeking clients' views. (See Mayer and Timms, 1970: 16.)

With the benefit of further thinking and developments in social work since the early 1970s we may add to this list. Most consumers of social work are working-class and are women. Many are black. Many are elderly. Significant numbers are unable to articulate responses to research instruments like questionnaires and structured interviews. It is perhaps for these reasons, too, that social work clients are not always considered as having credible opinions – even about their own lives and circumstances. Ann Oakley (1980), for example, tells the stories of encounters between women and doctors during pregnancy and childbirth. The experiences and understandings of women were discounted – even to the extent, for one woman, of contradicting her information as to how many children she had! The doctor is the expert.

Helen Kettleborough, in consultations on local authority services with women in Tameside, uncovered a wealth of ideas and suggestions about service provision. Local womens groups were contacted:

Common to all these women's groups is their lack of access to power, and to the local decision making processes. Women's groups do not represent a strong pressure group on the council. Whilst some women's groups might be seen as more acceptable than others, they are all characterised by a lack of influence and status when decisions are made. As a result, women's opinion of, for example, council services, are largely unknown. (Kettleborough, 1988: 57)

In ensuring that black as well as white women were consulted, the exercise revealed that services were not equally available to black women and communities and were hampered in their effectiveness through the lack of black and bilingual staff. All women, disabled and able-bodied, commented on the lack of access to public facilities. Disabled women suggested that improvements could be made in the provision of aids and adaptations (Kettleborough, 1988: 59–60). Consulting consumers does provide knowledge for the effective development of services.

Black people have been invisible as consumers of social services. It is only very recently that thought has been given by those in social welfare to the particular problems black people experience in a predominantly white society which discriminates against people because of the colour of their skin. Services have been provided with little or no attention to the importance of culture, custom, religion and language. Stereotypical assumptions are made about the lives of black people which lead to inappropriate and ineffective service delivery. For example, the King's Fund Centre study of carers in Afro-Caribbean, Asian and Chinese communities in Southwark found that many carers were unaware of the services that might be available to them. Additionally, service providers did not understand these carers' needs. They tended to make false assumptions about the support and help available to them through extended families (McCalman, 1990).

Researchers have been particularly neglectful in developing methods appropriate for eliciting information from people who may not be articulate in the English language. Little thought has been given to respondents who may not have the necessary language or verbal skills. Chapman and Green suggest that linking community work with research in action–research can bring benefit to research, in that 'community work knowledge and skills can provide privileged access to the experiences and views of people who are the subjects of that research' (Chapman and Green, 1990: 15).

Similarly social workers have skills in communicating with children and with people with mental, speech and hearing disabilities. Putting research and evaluation into the hands of practitioners should provide opportunities for ensuring that all consumers' views are sought.

But *The Client Speaks* was forward looking in many ways. It anticipated social work resources being in short supply and warned against the client being regarded as ' "sovereign" or an "economic man" who should be encouraged to "shop around" in a market of social services' (Mayer and Timms, 1970: 3). Having regard to empowerment and to being open to all perceptions of social work, it clearly is right to consult the consumer. Evidence suggests that an increasing number of social welfare organisations, both statutory and voluntary, now acknowledge this responsibility and recognise that consulting the consumer can enhance the effectiveness of services (Croft and Beresford 1990). To become 'consumerist', however, may present problems (Sainsbury, 1987). Consumers, like practitioners (and researchers) can be racist, sexist and intolerant. One only has to reflect on the strength of consumer opinion when it comes to plans, within policies of 'normalisation', to purchase a terraced house to provide a home for people with mental handicaps or to convert the large dilapidated Victorian house in the neighbourhood into a bail hostel. Consulting the consumer, in the name of participatory democracy, can be a mechanism to prevent change for equality and preserve the status quo.

Further, consumers of social services may have very low expectations of quality and resources. Clearly this has implications for understanding consumer views in the evaluation of welfare services. It is important that such evaluations are not used to ration services or to maintain quality at a level that neither the social worker nor the manager would tolerate themselves.

The professional task of the practitioner is to negotiate the meanings of views expressed:

> Client study researchers have tended to be stronger on moral prescription than on sociological theorizing. Their wish to give the client a good hearing has had a healthy and welcome impact on social work research and practice. But without an equal measure of social theory there is always the danger that understanding is sacrificed to reforming zeal. Asking clients to speak remains a fundamentally important research task. Adding theory to the client's view not only tells us how practice is experienced but also helps us to understand something of the nature of social work itself and the times in which it was formed. (Howe, 1990: 76)

David Howe argues for seeking the client's view but against both objectivist and subjectivist positions in relation to the meaning of what the client says. He shows that the way the consumer is viewed will influence what is heard and indeed what is said. 'The professional expert' (Mayer and Timms's psychoanalytic social worker), perhaps typified now in the early 1990s by the family therapist (Howe 1991), uses what the client says to contribute to the expert diagnosis of client pathology. In common with the dominant model of evaluation, 'the professional expert', as scientist and technicist, objectifies the client and takes utterances as indicators of behavioural variables and personal characteristics. Thus, in evaluation, a criticism of the therapist by the client may be interpreted as an indicator of resistance to treatment. The 'subjectivist', on the other hand, regards the clients' perceptions of their subjective experiences as the only valid knowledge. The subjectivist social worker attempts to understand the client's experience totally from the client's point of view, failing to understand the ways in which the client's perspective is constructed. The 'welfare manager' hears the client's view differently again:

> the client is defined, not in terms of some scientific theory or inter-subjective encounter, but by someone deciding what the other person shall mean . . . . For example, many clients of social workers are defined by law, that is by how they behave rather than why they behave. (Howe, 1990: 69)

The 'welfare manager' asks clients to speak in order to categorise them in relation to provision.

We share Howe's conclusion that this reveals the importance of epistemology in social work. To be locked into either objectivity or subjectivity is to be confined to partial understandings: 'Like the social scientist, the social worker is engaged in the study of social meaning and not in the search for an objective truth' (Howe, 1990: 70).

In the final part of this chapter we will explore ways in which the practitioner, in assuming responsibility for evaluation, may develop methods to reveal meanings of social work. First, we anticipate the emergence of a further model of evaluation – that related to inspection, performance review, monitoring and quality assurance.

An emerging paradigm: inspection, performance review, monitoring and quality assurance

The collection of official statistics in social welfare organisations might be understood as a form of monitoring the demands made upon organisations and the services delivered by them. In reality, however, official statistics have been collected for central government returns and rarely is use made of them within organisations to monitor their own policies and services. One example of more internal attempts to collect data for monitoring purposes has been in the implementation of equal opportunities staff recruitment and selection policies. This has been important. If policy change is taken seriously, then the organisation will need to know the extent of the effect of policy change on practice. The requirement itself to complete a monitoring form can contribute to the effective implementation of policy through raising awareness (see Connelly, 1989: 46).

Both the community care legislation (National Health Service and Community Care Act 1990) and the Children Act 1989 place emphasis on the development of systems for inspection and quality control (House of Commons 1990). The Department of Health circular on inspection units (DoH, 1990) recommends that local authorities establish inspection and quality control operations with advisory committees comprising representatives of the local authority, voluntary and private organisations, and consumers. Two features are emphasised: first, that inspection and quality control should operate consistently across local authorities; second, that inspection should be at 'arm's length' from the provision of services. The priority for inspection is to ensure standards in those organisations with which the local authority makes agreements for the provision of residential, day care and domiciliary care. Recognition is given, however, to the eventual extension of quality control to other areas.

Monitoring and arm's length inspection are both top-down mechanisms to check on the implementation of and adherence to standards in practice. They are important in terms of accountability and public scrutiny. A danger is that, in their structural and organisational separation from practice, systems of monitoring and inspection will be based on positivist epistemologies. Criteria of performance probably will be devised that can be measured through the collection of quantifiable data by means of standardised research instruments, such as questionnaires, forms and annual returns. Such models of inspection and quality control may not always check on bad practice. The history of quality control in relation to child protection services and residential care suggests that more qualitative and subjective data on performance will be collected and examined only when something goes wrong – and then in an inquisitorial context.

The relationship between monitoring and inspection on the one hand and quality on the other is complex. Every practitioner knows how data can be fudged, how routines develop around the completion of forms that may bear little relationship with what goes on in practice. The task of inspection and quality control in safeguarding standards must be twofold: to provide systems through which statutory, voluntary and private social welfare organisations are publicly accountable; and to ensure that services and practices are evaluated in such a way as to ensure good practice. The experience of data production for official statistics and monitoring generates a fear that bureaucratic systems will develop in ways meaningless to the development of day-to-day good practice. In the same way that the external evaluator adopting the dominant, positivist model of evaluation fails to impinge on practice, so this could also be the case if inspection relies on a similar model.

Practitioner evaluation is essential to good practice and to quality assurance. We hope that the emerging quality control and inspection units for social welfare will assure themselves that effective systems of evaluation are integrated with routine practices in social welfare organisations. It is often left to brave practitioners and brave users to comment on bad practice. To ensure that quality systems really work, they need to be empowered.

Also models of inspection in themselves may shape practice: 'Embedded within the dominant form of teacher evaluation is the assumption that teaching is a commodified product in which expert teachers deposit the "right" information into the heads of students' (Gitlin and Smyth, 1989: 25). At this stage we can only speculate about the relationship that may develop between inspectorial systems of performance review and quality assurance and particular commodified forms of social work practice which emphasise expert technique and case management. This form of evaluation will submerge questions about what is good practice and will legitimate particular forms of practice based on positivist techniques and supposed objectivity and neutrality.

The practitioner as evaluator

Finally in this chapter we explore possibilities for an evaluation model in which the practitioner takes responsibility for evaluating practice. Following the same format as preceding chapters, the elements of the model explored are its value base; its ethical position; the purposes of practitioner evaluation; communication of such evaluation; roles; and skills of the practitioner–evaluator.

Value base

Values are integral to evaluation. The very term contains the notion of value. The fundamental task in evaluation is to place value on an activity. Increasingly, in the new managerialism of social welfare, value is connected with the notion of cost, 'value-for-money' (see Kelly, 1991). The dominant positivist model of evaluation, in its adherence to the 'expert' view, copes with values by assuming that the 'expert' can neutralise them. It is assumed that objectives of the social programme, criteria for assessing the extent to which they are achieved, and input and performance, can be objectively analysed using research techniques. But for objectives, criteria and documents of practice to be presented as though value-free is to deny their fundamental relationship with values and accept as given the pervasiveness of dominant values in our society and culture. The professional practitioner to whom this book is addressed would constantly reflect on objectives, methods and practices in relation to the fundamental purposes – the direction – of the work.

Jeffs and Smith use the idea of 'direction' to conceptualise purpose, something which is broader than objectives and involves 'having a personal but shared idea of the "good": some notion of what makes for human flourishing and well-being' (Jeffs and Smith, 1990: 17). It is in relation to the 'direction' of the piece of work that professional judgements are made: about ethics, purposes, ways in which to communicate, about roles and appropriate skills. Social welfare practice cannot be made technical. It is complex and contradictory and informed with values at every stage in all its aspects. To make explicit the objectives of a particular piece of work is not enough. Objectives must be evaluated and reflected upon, reappraised, modified, fine-tuned and maybe rejected if they do not contribute to the direction of the work, to the overall and fundamental purpose.

The distinction between objective and direction, purpose, is important. An example to illustrate this is drawn from children's legislation. An overriding *objective* of child care practice in the 1960s and 1970s came to be the prevention of children being received into the care of the local authority. League tables were published comparing rates of admission to care (the criteria for measuring the extent to which the objective is achieved) of different local authorities and comparing area teams within each authority. The *objective* came to take the place of the *purpose*, the well-being and positive development of children. The 1980s brought with them a questioning of the 'prevention into care' *objective.* Social work practitioners began to argue for care as treatment and that to be received into care might provide an opportunity for the child to be appropriately treated. Treatment as an *objective* began to replace prevention. Perhaps one of the most radical aspects of the 1989 Children Act is that it requires us to reconsider the *purposes* of child care legislation, provision and practice before setting out on programmes to meet particular objectives. Purpose and action, theory and practice are integral to each other in the development of good practice. This is perhaps best summed up as follows:

Principles are the colours on the social worker painter's palette. The range and quality of colour helps to produce a good painting, but it is the painter's skill which makes or mars the picture. Excessive caseloads or the lack of necessary resources can be as disabling to the social worker as lack of paint to the artist, but failure to understand and apply essential principles can spoil even the best resources so that they become damaging to those they were intended to benefit. (DoH, 1989: 17)

The practitioner–evaluator, with colleagues, workers from other agencies, users and managers, will constantly ask 'What is the purpose of what we are doing?', 'What is the purpose of this service?' and 'What is the purpose of this group/programme project?'

The action–research model allows for the possibility of change, complexity, conflict and contradiction in the processes of social programmes. The consumer model lays emphasis on the client's, rather then the expert's, view. Both these models question fundamentally the notion of objectivity in evaluation and build in a recognition that subjective understandings differ. The client's view, the parents', the child's, the mother's, the father's, may all differ: so too that of the social workers, the health visitors, the police, the Director of Social Services, the councillors. One way to cope with different ideas and perceptions of the purposes, objectives and processes of social programmes is to allow for them all. The evaluator's task then could become one of making explicit these different views, leaving it to the readers of the report or the one who has commissioned the evaluation to make sense of the different views and judge between them.

Our approach, though, is to argue that the professional respons-ibility of the practitioner is to make judgements between competing views. In the previous chapter we outlined ideas for an ethical practice for the making of such judgements. The fundamental purpose of social welfare acts as the yardstick against which views are measured, sets the overall direction of the programme against which all other objectives and activities are understood. An example is drawn from a local community health project in which the regular women users complained about one afternoon of the project being reserved for Asian women. If one criterion for evaluation were based on the number of women using the centre, the expression of consumer dissatisfaction' combined with this criterion might then suggest that reserved times for Asian women be discontinued. These views would be understood by the practitioner–evaluator perhaps as an indication of the need for anti-racist training with the regular white users, as well as practitioners.

Ethics

Ethics must be considered in relation to purposes of evaluation, the ways in which evaluation is undertaken and data are collected, and the use and dissemination of evaluation findings. Ethics are complex and contradictory. For example, it is unethical to be covert (to hide) but ethical to respect confidentiality (to ensure that some information remains hidden from others). There is not the space in this chapter to analyse all aspects of ethics and ethical codes in relation to evaluation. Two ethical issues that are particularly relevant are the issue of being covert and the issue of pay, the piper and the tune!

When to hide and when not to hide relates to all stages of practice evaluation. The issue may relate to hiding theories and assumptions, hiding the fact that data are being collected and hiding findings. Evaluation is to do with teasing out, making explicit, assumptions, concepts and theories that inform practice – that lead to decisions to intervene in people's lives or to deliver some services in preference to others. The ethics of when and how this is done and with whom is a matter of professional judgement with regard to the direction of the work. Hiding from people the fact that data are being collected is unethical. But the distinction between hiding and revealing is complex: are research purposes and uses of findings hidden if the respondent does not fully understand explanations that have been given? In both social research and social work practice covert observation is sometimes undertaken. The practitioner–evaluator appraised of ethical debates in research would develop a consciousness of the ownership of knowledge and information. For example, because the practitioner–evaluator is not an outside, objective 'expert', she is likely to gather sensitive information through informal contacts and networks, observing their colleague at the next desk, or hearing the gossip in the pub. Framing such information in research terms can provide ways of addressing the complexity and ethics of using such information.

Another ethical difficulty with respect to honesty arises from the political context of evaluation. The oversimplified ethical position in relation to research findings is that they should not be hidden. But widespread publication of findings that cast doubt on a particular social programme when, at the same time, there are attempts by the funding authority to reduce budgets may not be the most effective way of continuing with the programme and pursuing the direction of the work, albeit with changes and modifications arising from evaluation.

'He who pays the piper calls the tune.' In the introductory chapter we stressed the need for the professional practitioner to be autonomous of both bureaucracy and profession. We argued that being research-minded should enable the practitioner to work in this way: to develop methods of systematic analysis and reason to counter traditional, taken-for-granted routine practices and even actively to resist instruction. It is not in the interests of good practice for 'he' who pays the practitioner to call the tune. So too with the practitioner as evaluator. Indeed one of the very reasons not to invest management with total responsibility for inspection and quality control (as the Social Services Inspectorate does in its guidance [DoH/SSI 1991]) is to ensure that resource and fiscal matters do not skew evaluation findings and their presentation. So it is inappropriate for the local authority which grant-aids the voluntary project to evaluate it, although quite appropriate for it to require that the funded work be evaluated. Equally, it is inappropriate for the voluntary project to skew its findings to match the criteria for the next budget round. Evaluators must resist playing the tune they think the piper wants to hear whilst at the same time being mindful that evaluation findings are knowledge and knowledge is power.

Purposes

The purpose of practitioner evaluation is to reflect critically on the effectiveness of personal and professional practice. Such practice cannot be evaluated out of context. Practice is historically and culturally constructed and takes place within social, political and economic contexts. Practice is also conducted with others: with managers, with other workers, with users and members of the community. In the evaluation of the effectiveness of social programmes, policy, services and personnel, power cannot be divorced from practice. The dominant model of evaluation isolates practice from context. Its over riding concern is with performance indicators and behavioural outcomes. Context and power remain implicit, uncontested and not open to question, analysis and change. Inspection and quality assurance, if based on such a model (as it has been in teacher evaluation), will focus on gathering evidence on practitioner performance to ensure 'correct' practice. Evaluation as inspection becomes part of the surveillance and control of practitioners within existing structures and patterns of power. Practitioners who are socialised within such a model and comply may, in turn, engage in the surveillance and control of people with whom they work: 'the contrast is between the managerial relations of inspection, domination and quality control, versus the educative relations of collegiality, reflection and empowerment' (Gitlin and Smyth, 1989: 42).

The purpose of evaluation in practice is to contribute to development of 'good' rather than 'correct' practice (Jeffs and Smith 1990). Similarly, Gitlin and Smyth use the concept of 'rightness':

> Missing from the instrumental and technicist ways of evaluating teaching are the kinds of educative relationships that permit the asking of moral, ethical and political questions about the 'rightness' of actions. When based upon educative (as distinct from managerial) relations, evaluative practices become concerned with breaking down structured silences and narrow prejudices. (Gitlin and Smyth, 1989: 161)

Evaluation becomes concerned with making visible what goes on in practice. Its purpose is not simply to test whether narrowly defined objectives have been met. It is continually to question and problematise definitions of social need and established responses by social welfare agencies to that need. Further, it is to understand and make explicit the impact of economic and social policies and structures on the chances of practice moving in the direction of the 'good'.

Communication

Fundamental to a model of practitioner evaluation is communication. Jeffs and Smith (1990) and Gitlin and Smyth (1989) advocate dialogue as the means by which practitioners can, with others, be critically reflective. Dialogue involves 'the critical testing of pre-judgements that empowers the actor to challenge the taken-for-granted notions that influence the way they see the world and judge their practice' (Gitlin and Smyth, 1989: 4).

Dialogical communication for evaluation does not only take place between colleagues, but with all actors in the situation, with users, managers and workers from other agencies – within the 'community of inquirers'. Communication is not an end in itself but a means by which prejudices, assumptions and stereotypical concepts can be drawn out, our own and others: not to accord validity to them in their own right as commodities, but to subject them to theoretical and empirical analysis. It is important not simply to provide opportunities for words to be spoken. Finding ways to enable us to understand is crucial: to understand what we are saying, why and how we come to be saying such things, and the effect of naming and labelling on how we understand the world.

Gitlin and Smyth (1989) use the term 'dialogical evaluation'. For communication and debate to become dialogical evaluation, inter-personal power and the power of dominant discourses in naming the social world have to be addressed. Power does not only operate hierarchically. It is not enough to argue that the practitioner, in taking responsibility for evaluation, will work for the 'good' in contrast to the hierarchical manager who has only a conception of the 'correct'. Power operates through the structural organisation of social welfare departments and their day-to-day routines, proce-dures and methods of work. Thus Foucault (1980) argues that analyses of power are fruitless if obsessed with who is thought to possess the power. Rather, what is crucial is to be aware of, to observe, analyse and understand power in action, in practice, in key decision making and in nondecision-making processes (the proces-ses that ensure that some issues are prevented from becoming visible, some questions are not asked) (Bachrach and Baratz, 1970). This analysis of interpersonal power can be extended to include aspects of power such as style, language, gestures and image. The dialogical method is thus one concerned with the way power operates and its intended and unintended consequences for 'good' practice. (See Silverman, 1985, for an explanation of Foucault's work and its application in qualitative research.)

Roles

The fundamental role of the practitioner–evaluator is to engage in and facilitate dialogue. Thus the role is not only as evaluator of personal practice but as facilitator and enabler to ensure that others significant to the practice have the same opportunity. This means that the role might be conceived, in part, as one of educator, providing opportunities for others: to develop skills in analysis, reflection and debate; to have the confidence to assert that their knowing of the world is relevant, and to be prepared to be self-critical, to reject cherished and long-held ideas; to be passionate but at the same time tentative about what is the problem, what should be done.

The practitioner would have particular regard for those who historically have had little say in what happens to them in their own lives, those oppressed through interpersonal, institutional and structural processes. Such people, who may express their views through anger, would be listened to and both understood and encouraged themselves to understand. They would not be labelled as difficult (Cain, 1989). Similarly, but in contrast, the practitioner has responsibility to engage with those in managerial positions to encourage them into the 'community of inquirers', according them the opportunity to reflect critically on practice and the delivery of services, having regard to the fundamental and overall purposes of social welfare and the direction of the work, releasing them from preoccupation with departmental objectives and routines.

Skills

The skills of practitioner evaluation are those of data collection, analysis, theoretical reflection and development, recording and report writing. These skills are well documented in research methods texts.

Gitlin and Smyth usefully explore the skills necessary to engage in dialogical evaluation. These skills relate to argument, reason and debate and are necessary to problematise practice, to observe it and provide accounts of it (Gitlin and Smyth, 1989: 98). The conditions necessary for the practitioner–evaluator are, first, that no participant in the evaluation has prior claim to being right and, second, that it must be accepted by all participants that perceptions are always partial, may indeed be mistaken, and that dialogue is the means through which more valid and reliable understandings can emerge. We would add further conditions. Practice, particular interventions, services, methods and programmes, must always be held as tentative knowing that they may be wrong, ineffective or discriminatory. Practitioner–evaluators must be constantly uncertain about what they are doing and about social strategies embarked upon. Evaluation is to do with change, not defence.

The process of dialogical evaluation starts with an analysis of intention and practice, an examination of practice with regard to the intended direction of the work. Contradictions between intentions and practices will emerge that can then be explored for their meaning. Intentions as well as practices are tentative. Through critical reflection and dialogue alternatives will emerge which are important to the development and change for 'good' practice. Asking difficult and challenging questions of each other, and of the policies, procedures and routines within the organisation, will make visible the choices that have been made between alternatives. This will open up our personal and historical biographies and organisational practices, and expose the relationships between the personal, our ideas, not only how we see and understand the world but also how we intervene in it. Thus, 'commonsense', taken-for-granted routine practices, through which power operates and inequalities are maintained, become subject to personal and public scrutiny. Knowledge of practice is generated for the practitioner and others involved in the practice rather than for the outside 'expert' and the relationship between knowledge, action and change becomes dynamic.

9

Conclusion

We set out in this book to explore some ways in which certain types of research methodologies may be retrieved to inform social work methodologies. We passionately believed that the practice-versus-research traditions in social work could be dismantled through the development of new kinds of critical, reflective practice. By this we mean particular ways of thinking about social work theory and practice, such as:

● the questioning of taken-for-granted assumptions about the definition of problems and the categorisation of need;
● recognising the ways in which ideas, thoughts, understandings and opinions are shaped historically, economically, politically and socially through social structures and processes;
● making the implicit explicit;
● raising the profile of value positions and working with the problematics they generate;
● locating practice in its agency contexts so that service delivery issues are not addressed as routine constraints;
● building reflection, involvement and evaluation into every stage of the practice process.

Practitioners have often experienced research as alienating, irrelevant and exploitative because they have been treated as 'objects' in the process. This is the very antithesis of the type of approach we have tried to unravel and develop in this book. There are many political, historical and professional reasons for such 'objectification'. These can be summarised in one way by saying that social work's disengagement from research is a disengagement from positivism. Accordingly, it was necessary in the book to question the 'taken-for-grantedness' of different epistemologies, including positivism.

In Chapter 2, we attempted to demonstrate the importance of epistemology to social work. By referring to psychodynamic, Marxist and feminist theoretical perspectives in social work, we illustrated how different ways of knowing and understanding the world make different assumptions about the individual and society and their interrelationship. We drew attention to the ways in which power operates through ways of knowing. To have the right to know, and to know about, others and to have the right to intervene on the basis of this knowledge is powerful. In practice that is emancipatory these issues need to be addressed. Reflecting on claims to know made in psychodynamic, Marxist and feminist theories, we came to a number of conclusions. They all offer perspectives that should be seen as not necessarily competing but complementary to inform social work. Theory and research are distinguished from common sense in that they construct everyday, taken-for-granted concepts theoretically in order critically to appraise them. Theory is never certain. It only provides 'good enough' explanations and understandings until something better comes along. Research-minded practitioners need to be passionate in what they do, but also tentative and uncertain.

In developing our thinking in this way we came to share a particular stance on the purposes and values of research. This stance affirmed the importance of subjectivity, social context and the valuing of people. This contrasts sharply with the objectifying tradition of research. We believe that, if practitioners can find an alternative relationship with research, 'own it' and make it compatible with social work values, then quite new possibilities are opened up. More acceptable forms of enquiry can become inalienable parts of the repertoire of the practitioner who is research-minded. The values underlying practice that is research-minded include:

● acknowledging that everyone has skills, ability and understanding;
● respecting people's rights and bases for reciprocity;
● appreciating the complexities in problems of living;
● knowing that people acting collectively can be powerful;
● practising what one preaches;
● challenging all forms of oppression.

If research in social work can become an integral part of practice, then living out these values can empower every participant in the process.

These broad-brush themes about critical reflective practice, epistemologies and values brought us to the door of a methodology for research-minded practice. What would it look like? We began to explore the possibilities by examining issues to be addressed at every stage of the process: preparation and groundwork; problem formulation; data collection and analysis; evaluation. We began to realise that our approach was not necessarily compatible with every type of practice. For example, the values we espouse indicate a developmental model of welfare which gives priority to such things as:

● accessible, localised services;
● proactive approaches to locally identified needs;
● self-help and networking;
● advocacy;
● participation of users in service development.

We then realised that we were developing a model of research-minded practice informed by the methodologies and experiences of participatory research. Values underlying empowerment come to shape purposes such as the development of anti-oppressive practices. Communication becomes open rather than closed, so that ownership and understanding of values, knowledge and skills are shared. Participants in the process develop reciprocal roles as partners and enablers, within 'communities of inquirers', so that skills are used to empower rather than to deskill or alienate members. Participation and reciprocal relations are contextualised and theorised to take account of power.

It became evident that, as we were struggling to make explicit the assumptions underlying the model of research-minded practice we were attempting to develop, the problematic of that model had to be addressed. Social work cannot always be based fully upon developmental and participatory principles because it is also practised in contexts which embrace quite different values and power bases such as those of social control. It is easy to see how issues like confidentiality have to be negotiated rather differently in this context. The point about practitioners who are research-minded is that they will 'own' and address these issues in a value-based manner rather than bury or hide them in the backyard of practice wisdom or elitist expertise. Furthermore, the prospects for negotiating developmental principles in less developmental contexts will be addressed. Social work has always had to carry out its mission in relation to the political economy of the age and this is no less true of applied research for better practice. This will be shown to be so as research-minded practitioners begin their journeys of critical reflection in relation to the Children Act 1989, 'Care in the Community' and 'Punishment in the Community'.

Formulating the issues in practice proved to be an illuminating area in which to open up prospects for retrieving and reclaiming some research traditions in social work. We found that some research reports and literature on practice theory share the view that assessment in social work involves an active and complex process of conceptualisation as practitioners socially construct their worlds. Research-minded practitioners do not approach this task as a narrowly defined technical exercise: their thinking starts a long way back in the process. Ethical, political, policy and practice issues are actively questioned even in relation to the very decision to engage or not to engage with this person, in this way, in joint, reciprocal formulations of problems. No entry is always an option, and the implications of missing data are thought through in terms of agency constructions rather than technical deficiencies. Role induction is seen as a mutual process of education and empowerment as practitioners skilfully engage with participants.

We see these value-based practices as just as appropriate and possible as research-minded practitioners engage with subjects to generate data. If data are the building-blocks of research and practice, then the ethics of giving and receiving data must be subject to critical scrutiny and reflection. This means that practitioners need to engage carefully and critically with others in negotiation about what is admissible knowledge. Data collection is a process of active and reciprocal exchange between all participants: it is not a matter of passive responses to a predetermined set of questions. Again, the data collection process itself should express values about rights, reciprocity, empowerment and anti-oppressive practices.

To be understood data need to be analysed. Analysis is an ongoing process throughout all stages of practice, moving back and forth between data and theory. It is a process in which participants engage dialogically. Analysis is the process of negotiating meaning. The practitioner's responsibility in this is to ensure that all have opportunity in this process and to make judgements between competing views. That research often looks down, presenting the view from above, was reflected on. The research-minded practitioner would have particular regard for the view from below, according credibility to those who are often unheard, providing an opportunity for them to reflect on ways in which their views have been shaped in a society of inequality.

We noted with interest that evaluations in social work have always been informed by research methodologies, but, even here, the same story can be told. Evaluation has often suffered from the limits of positivism, such as experimental designs and epidemiological surveys. Furthermore, evaluation as part of the social work process has not necessarily been enhanced by research methodologies. It is often undertaken by practitioners in a relatively perfunctory and rudimentary manner or in response to management demands. Evaluative studies have also been sometimes used to disparage social workers by considering their practices in decontextualised ways: driving a further nail into the coffin of applied research for better practice!

The practitioner–evaluator can, however, embrace the methodologies outlined:

- the value base acknowledges change, complexity, conflict and contradiction in social work;
- ethics indicate the need to be explicit about purposes and to respect the boundaries of permitted and required endeavour and involvement;
- communication between all participants is dialogical, a process of exploring each other's subjective perceptions and evaluations and understanding the historical, structural and cultural influences on these views;
- the practitioner is a partner, enabler, facilitator and educator;
- skills are those of the good practitioner – openness, honesty, thoughtfulness, clear thinking and critical reflection.

As we reach the end of our journey, we realise that we have only just started it. It will be apparent that we have not achieved a definitive methodology for the research-minded practitioner. We have omitted detailed consideration of the organisational contexts of practice. What is a research-minded organisation? How can the practitioner negotiate the methodologies outlined in the contexts of contemporary welfare and penal agencies? Our hope is that we have begun to open up the way to exploring new possibilities for research and practice to be brought together to enhance the lives of people living in oppressive and vulnerable circumstances. The path is not clear and there are no safe hiding places. But it is worthwhile embarking on this journey if we are committed to the values we have steadfastly tried to embrace through our work for this book.

Bibliography

Addison, C. and Rosen, G. (1985) 'Practice Research in a Social Services Department', in P. Wedge (ed.), *Social Work – Research into Practice, Proceedings of the First Annual JUC/BASW Conference*, Birmingham, BASW Publications.

Ahmed, S. (1989) 'Research and the Black Experience', in M. Stein (ed.), *Research into Practice: Proceedings of the Fourth Annual JUC/BASW Conference*, Leeds University, Birmingham, BASW Publications.

Ahmed, S., Cheetham, J. and Small, J. (1986) *Social Work with Black Children and their Families*, London, Batsford.

Ali, S. (1991) *The Needs of Asian Elders in Newcastle*, Report of a study commissioned by Search, Newcastle, with the Social Welfare Research Unit, Newcastle Polytechnic.

Althusser, L. (1971) *Lenin, Philosophy and Other Essays*, London, New Left Books.

Archer, J. L. and Whitaker, D. S. (1989) 'Engaging Practitioners in Formulating Research Purposes', *Social Work Education* 8 (2), Spring, 29–37.

Attlee, C. (1920) *The Social Worker*, London, Bell.

Bachrach, P. and Baratz, M.S. (1970) *Power and Poverty, Theory and Practice*, New York, Oxford University Press.

Bailey, R. and Lee, P. (eds) (1982) *Theory and Practice in Social Work*, Oxford, Blackwell.

Baker, R. (1976) 'The Multirole Practitioner in the Generic Orientation to Social Work Practice', *British Journal of Social Work*, vol. 6, no. 3, 327–52.

Ball, C., Harris, R., Roberts, G. and Vernon, S. (1988) *The Law Report: Teaching and Assessment of Law in Social Work Education*, Paper 4.1, London, Central Council for Education and Training in Social Work.

Becker, H. S. (1970) 'Whose side are we on?', in J. D. Douglas (ed.), *The Relevance of Sociology*, New York, Appleton-Century Crofts.

Berger, P. and Luckmann, T. (1971) *The Social Construction of Reality*, Harmondsworth, Penguin.

Bocock, R. (1988) 'Psychoanalysis and Social Theory', in G. Pearson, J. Treseder and M. Yelloly (eds), *Social Work and the Legacy of Freud*, Basingstoke, Macmillan Education.

140   *Bibliography*

Booth, T. (1988) *Developing Policy Research*, Aldershot, Avebury.
Brearley, J. (1991) 'A Psychodynamic Approach to Social Work', in J. Lishman (ed.), *Handbook of Theory for Practice Teachers in Social Work*, London, Jessica Kingsley.
Brook, E. and Davis, A. (1985) *Women, the Family and Social Work*, London, Tavistock.
Bulmer, M., Lewis, J., and Piachaud, D. (eds) (1989) *The Goals of Social Policy*, London, Unwin Hyman.
Burgess, R. G. (1984) *In the Field: An Introduction to Field Research*, London, George Allen & Unwin.
Cain, M. (ed.) (1989) *Growing Up Good: policing the behaviour of girls in Europe*, London, Sage.
Cain, M. and Smart, C. (1990) 'Foreword' to A. Worrall, *Offending Women: Female Lawbreakers and the Criminal Justice System*, London, Routledge.
Campbell, D. T. (1979) 'Degrees of Freedom', and the Case Study in T. D. Cook and C. S. Reichardt (eds), *Qualitative and Quantitative Methods in Evaluation Research*, Beverly Hills, California and London, Sage.
Carby, H. (1982) 'White women listen! Black feminism and the boundaries of sisterhood', *The Empire Strikes Back*, edited by Centre for Contemporary Cultural Studies, London, Hutchinson.
Carew, R. (1979) 'The place of knowledge in social work', *British Journal of Social Work*, vol.9, no.3, 349–64.
Carr, W. and Kemmis, S. (1986) *Becoming Critical: Education, Knowledge and Action Research*, Lewes, Falmer.
CCETSW (1989) *Requirements and Regulations for the Diploma in Social Work DipSW*, Paper 30, London, Central Council for Education and Training in Social Work.
CCETSW/PSSC (1980) *Research and Practice, report of a working party on a research strategy for the personal social services*, London, Central Council for Education and Training in Social Work.
Chapman, A. and Green, J. (1990) 'The Lessons of the Community Development Project for Community Development Today', Paper no. 6, *Roots and Branches: A Winter School on Community Development and Health*, Health Education Authority and The Open University.
Cigno, K. (1988) 'Consumer views of a family centre drop-in', *British Journal of Social Work*, 18, 361–75.
Cohen, S. (1975) 'It's all right for you to talk: political and sociological manifestos for social work action', in R. Bailey and M. Brake (eds), *Radical Social Work*, London, Edward Arnold.
Connelly, N. (1989) *Race and Change in Social Services Departments*, London, Policy Studies Institute.
Corrigan, P. and Leonard, P. (1978) *Social Work Practice Under Capitalism: A Marxist Approach*, London, Macmillan.
Cousins, C. (1987) *Controlling Social Welfare; a sociology of state welfare work and organisation*, Brighton, Wheatsheaf.
Croft, S. and Beresford, P. (1984) 'Patch and Participation; the case for citizen research', *Social Work Today*, 17 September.
Croft, S. and Beresford, P. (1989) 'Listening to the Voice of the Consumer:

A New Model for Social Services Research', in M. Stein (ed.), *Research into Practice: Proceedings of the Fourth Annual JUC/BASW Conference,* Leeds University, Birmingham, BASW.

Croft, S. and Beresford, P. (1990) *From Paternalism to Participation: involving people in social services,* Open Services Project and Joseph Rowntree Foundation, London.

Curnock, K. and Hardiker, P. (1979) *Towards Practice Theory: Skills and Methods in Social Assessments,* London, Routledge & Kegan Paul.

Dale, J. and Foster, P. (1986) *Feminists and State Welfare,* London, Routledge & Kegan Paul.

Davis, K. O. (1990) 'Word-Power! The Academic Route to Power and Action!', *DCDP News,* Issue 39, 15–16, Clay Cross Derbyshire, Derbyshire Coalition of Disabled People.

Dean, R. G. and Fenby, B. L. (1989) 'Exploring epistemologies: social work action as a reflection of philosophical assumptions', *Journal of Social Work Education,* 25, 1, 46–54.

Department of Health (1989) *The Care of Children: Principles and Practice in Regulations and Guidance,* London, HMSO.

Department of Health/Social Services Inspectorate (1991) *Inspecting for Quality: guidance on practice for inspection units in social services departments and other agencies; principles, issues and recommendations,* London, HMSO.

Department of Health and Social Security (1985) *Social Work Decisions in Child Care,* London, HMSO.

Deutsch, S. E. and Howard, J. (1970) *Where It's At: Radical Perspectives in Sociology,* London, Harper & Row.

Dillon, R. (1990) *Report of the Action Project into Ethnically Sensitive Social Work,* Birmingham, BASW.

Dominelli, L. (1988) *Anti-Racist Social Work,* London, Macmillan.

Dominelli, L. and McLeod, E. (1989) *Feminist Social Work,* Basingstoke, Macmillan.

du Bois, B. (1983) 'Passionate Scholarship: notes on values, knowing and method in feminist social science', in G. Bowles and R. Duelli Klein (eds), *Theories of Women's Studies,* London, Routledge & Kegan Paul.

Duelli Klein, R. (1983) 'How To Do What We Want To Do: Thoughts About Feminist Methodology', in G. Bowles and R. Duelli Klein (eds), *Theories of Women's Studies,* London and New York, Routledge & Kegan Paul.

Dunne, T. P and Power, A. (1990) 'Sexual abuse and handicap: preliminary findings of a community based study', *Mental Handicap Research,* 3, 2.

Dutt, R. (1989) 'Griffiths Really is a White Paper', *Social Work Today* 21 (13), 23rd November, 34.

Dutt, R. (1990) 'Patronising White Attitude on Trans-racial Adoption', letter to *Social Work Today,* 21 (25), 1 March, 11.

Everitt, A. (1982) 'Research in CQSW Courses', Paper for CCETSW Workshop on Research-Related Skills for Social Work Students, 13/14 December, London, Central Council for Education and Training in Social Work, mimeo.

142   *Bibliography*

Everitt, A. (1990) 'Will Women Managers Save Social Work?', in P. Carter, T. Jeffs and M. Smith (eds), *Social Work and Social Welfare Yearbook 2*, Milton Keynes, Open University Press.

Everitt, A., Hardiker, P., Littlewood, J. and Mullender, A. (1991) 'Practitioner Research', Research and Changing Services for Children and Adults, Papers from the 6th Annual Joint University Council, Social Work Education Committee Research Conference, *Social Work and Social Sciences Review*, Supplement to Volume 3, 15–22.

Fay, B. (1975) *Social Theory & Political Practice*, London, George Allen & Unwin.

Feuerstein, M.-T. (1986) *Partners in Evaluation: Evaluating Development and Community Programmes with Participants*, London, Macmillan.

Filstead, W. J. (1979) 'Qualitative Methods: A Needed Perspective in Evaluation Research', in T. D. Cook and C. S. Reichardt (eds), *Qualitative and Quantitative Methods in Evaluation Research*, Beverly Hills, California and London, Sage.

Finch, J. (1984) 'It's Great to Have Someone to Talk to', in C. Bell and H. Roberts (eds), *Social Researching: Politics, Problems, Practice*, London, Routledge & Kegan Paul.

Finch, J. (1986) *Research and Policy: the uses of qualitative methods in social and educational research*, Lewes, Falmer.

Finch, J. and Groves, D. (1980) 'Community Care and the Family: A Case for Equal Opportunities', *Journal of Social Policy*, 9, 4.

Finch, J. and Groves, D. (1983) *The Labour of Love: Women, Work and Caring*, London, Routledge & Kegan Paul.

Fisher, M., Marsh, P. and Phillips, D., with Sainsbury, E. (1986) *In and Out of Care: The Experiences of Children, Parents and Social Workers*, London, Batsford.

Foucault. M. (1979) *Discipline and Punish*, Harmondsworth, Penguin.

Foucault, M. (1980) *Power/Knowledge*, C. Gordon (ed.) New York, Pantheon.

Fruin, D. (1980) *Data Analysis: a basic introduction*, National Institute for Social Work papers no. 11, London, NISW.

Fruin, D. (1987) 'Book Review – Leaving Care by M. Stein and K. Carey', *British Journal of Social Work*, 17, 555–7.

Fuss, D. (1989) *Essentially Speaking: Feminism, Nature and Difference*, London, Routledge.

Galper, J. (1975) *The Politics of Social Service*, Englewood Cliffs, NJ, Prentice-Hall.

Giddens, A. (1989) *Sociology*, Cambridge, Polity Press.

Gitlin, A. and Smyth, J. (1989) *Teacher Evaluation: Educative Alternatives*, London, Falmer.

Glaser, B. and Strauss, A.L. (1967) *The Discovery of Grounded Theory*, Chicago, Aldine Publishing Co.

Goldberg, M. (1970) *Helping the Aged*, London, George Allen & Unwin.

Goldberg, M. (1972) 'The Use of Research in Social Work Education', Paper delivered to the XVIth International Congress of Schools of Social

Work, The Hague, in *New Themes in Social Work Education*, International Association of Schools of Social Work, New York, 1973.

Gosling, J. (1990) *A Model for User Consultation: the processes of involving service users with disabilities in planning, delivery and evaluation of services to them*, People for People Forum, Princes House, 32 Park Row, Nottingham, NG1 6GR.

Gouldner, A. (1971) *The Coming Crisis of Western Sociology*, London, Heinemann.

Habermas, J. (1974) *Theory and Practice*, London, Heinemann.

Halsey, A. H. (ed.) (1972) *Educational Priority, Vol. 1: EPA Problems and Policies*, Report of a research project sponsored by the Department of Education and Science and the Social Science Research Council, London, Department of Education and Science, HMSO.

Hammersley, M. and Atkinson, P. (1983) *Ethnography: Principles in Practice*, London, Tavistock.

Hanmer, J. and Statham, D. (1988) *Women and Social Work: Towards a Women-Centred Practice*, London, Macmillan.

Hanscombe, G. E. and Forster, J. (1982) *Rocking the Cradle: Lesbian Mothers, a challenge in family living*, London, Sheba Feminist Publishers.

Hanvey, C. (1990) 'Through a glass clearly', *Community Care*, 24 May, 23–4.

Hardiker, P. (1989) 'The Organisation and Management of Postgraduate Research Projects', University of Leicester, Faculty of the Social Sciences PhD Programme, mimeo.

Hardiker, P. and Barker, M. (eds) (1981) *Theories of Practice in Social Work*, London, Academic Press.

Hardiker, P. and Barker, M. (1986) *A Window on Child Care Practices in the 1980s*, University of Leicester, School of Social Work Research Report.

Hardiker, P. and Barker, M. (1991) 'Towards Social Theory for Social Work', in J. Lishman (ed.), *Handbook of Theory for Practice Teachers in Social Work*, London, Jessica Kingsley.

Hardiker, P., Exton, K. and Barker, M. (1989) *Policies and Practices in Preventive Child Care*, Report to the Department of Health, Leicester, University of Leicester.

Harding, S. (ed.) (1987) *Feminism and Methodology*, Indiana, Indiana University Press, and Milton Keynes, Open University Press.

Harris, J. (1989) 'The Webbs, The Charity Organisation Society and the Ratan Tata Foundation: Social policy from the perspective of 1912', in M. Bulmer, J. Lewis and D. Piachaud (eds), *The Goals of Social Policy*, London, Unwin Hyman.

Harwin, J. (1990) 'Parental responsibilities in the Children Act 1989', in N. Manning and C. Ungerson (eds), *Social Policy Review 1989–1990*, London, Longman.

Hearn, J. and Parkin, W. (1987) *'Sex at Work': The Power and Paradox of Organisation Sexuality*, Brighton, Wheatsheaf.

Heron, J. (1981) 'Philosophical Basis for a New Paradigm', in P. Reason and J. Rowan (eds), *Human Inquiry: A Sourcebook of New Paradigm Research*, Chichester, John Wiley & Sons.

Hogg, B., Kent, P. and Ward, D., (1990) 'Is there a right answer?', *Community Care*, no. 824, 26 July, 15.

Holman, R. (1970) 'Social work research today', in *Research and Social Work*, BASW Monograph no.4, London, 5–18.

Holman, R. (1987) 'Research from the Underside', *British Journal of Social Work*, 17, 669–83.

Holman, R. (1988) 'Research from the Underside', *Community Care*, 18 February, no. 699, 24–6.

Home Office (1986) *The Ethnic Origins of Prisoners*, London, HMSO.

House of Commons (1984) *Children in Care*, vol. 1, Second Report from the Social Services Committee Session 1983–84, London, HMSO.

House of Commons (1990) *Quality: report of the Social Services Committee*, London, HMSO.

Howe, D. (1987) *An Introduction to Social Work Theory*, Aldershot, Wildwood House and Community Care.

Howe, D. (1990) 'The Client's View in Context', in P. Carter, T. Jeffs and M. Smith (eds), *Social Work and Social Welfare Yearbook 2*, Buckingham, Open University Press.

Howe, D. (1991) 'Knowledge, Power and the Shape of Social Work Practice', in M. Davies (ed.), *The Sociology of Social Work*, London, Routledge.

Huxley, P. (1988) 'Quantitative-descriptive articles in the British Journal of Social Work volumes 1–14', *British Journal of Social Work*, 18 (2) April, 189–99.

Illich, I., McKnight, J., Zola, I. K., Caplan, J. and Shaiken, H. (1977) *The Disabling Professions*, London, Marion Boyers.

In Need Implementation Group (1991) *The Children Act and Children's Needs: Make It the Answer – not the Problem*, London, NCVO.

INODEP Ecumenical Institute for the Development of People (1981) *Conscientizing Research: a methodological guide*, Hong Kong, Plough Publications.

Irvine, E. (1969) 'Education for Social Work: Science or Humanity', *Social Work*, 26, 4, 3–6.

Jaehnig, W. (1973) 'Seeking out the disabled', in K. Jones (ed.), *The Year Book of Social Policy in Britain 1972*, London, Routledge & Kegan Paul.

Jeffs, T. and Smith, M. (eds) (1987) *Youth Work*, London, Macmillan.

Jeffs, T. and Smith, M. (1990) *Using Informal Education*, Buckingham, Open University Press.

Kahan, B. (1989) *Child Care Research, Policy and Practice*, London, Hodder & Stoughton.

Kelly, A. (1991) 'The 'New', Managerialism in the Social Services', in P. Carter, T. Jeffs and M. Smith (eds), *Social Work and Social Welfare Yearbook 3*, Buckingham, Open University Press.

Kemmis, S., 'Introduction', in S. Kemmis *et al.* (eds) (1984) *The Action Research Reader*, second edition, Victoria, Deakin University Press.

Kettleborough, H. (1988) 'Consulting Women in the Community about Local Government Services', in *Critical Social Policy*, issue 21, Spring, 56–67.

Kingsley, S. (1985) *Action Research: Method or Ideology?*, Wivenhoe, Essex, Association of Researchers in Voluntary Action and Community Involvement.

Langan, M. (1985) 'The unitary approach: a feminist critique', in E. Brook and A. Davis (eds), *Women, the Family and Social Work*, London, Tavistock Publications.

Langan, M. and Day, L. (eds) (1992) *Women, Oppression and Social Work* London, HarperCollins Academic.

Leissner, A., Herdman, K.A.M. and Davies, E.V. (1971) *Advice, Guidance and Assistance: a study of seven family advice centres*, London, Longman.

Leonard, P. (1975) 'Explanation and Education in Social Work', *British Journal of Social Work*, vol. 5, no. 3.

Leonard, P. (1984) *Personality and Ideology: Towards a Materialist Understanding of the Individual*, London, Macmillan.

Lorde, A. (1984) *Sister Outsider: Essays and Speeches*, New York, Crossing Press.

Lukes, S. (1974) *Power: a radical view*, London and Basingstoke, Macmillan.

McCalman, J. (1990) *The Forgotten People: Carers in three minority ethnic communities in Southwark*, London, King's Fund.

McTaggart, R. and the Curriculum Research Course Team (1982) *The Action Research Planner*, Victoria, Deakin University Press.

Mama, A. (1989) 'Violence against black women: Gender, race and state responses', *Feminist Review*, no. 32, 30–48.

Marris, P. and Rein, M. (1967) *Dilemmas of Social Reform*, London, Routledge & Kegan Paul.

Mayer, J.E. and Timms, N. (1970) *The Client Speaks: Working Class Impressions of Casework*, London, Routledge & Kegan Paul.

Meikle, J. (1988) 'Nottingham Advocacy Group: An Evaluation', unpublished.

Menzies Lyth, I. (1988) *Containing Anxiety in Institutions*, London, Free Association Books.

Meyer, H.J., Borgatta, E.F. and Jones, W.C. (1965) *Girls at Vocational High: an experiment in social work intervention*, New York, Russell Sage Foundation.

Mies, M. (1983) 'Towards a methodology for feminist research', in G. Bowles and R. Duelli Klein (eds), *Theories of Women's Studies*, London, Routledge & Kegan Paul.

Mills, C.W. (1959) *The Sociological Imagination*, New York, Oxford University Press.

Mills, C.W. (1963) 'On knowledge and power', in I.L. Horowitz (ed.), *Power, Politics and People: the collected essays of C.Wright Mills*, London, Oxford University Press.

Mishra, R. (1989) 'The academic tradition in social policy: The Titmus Years', in M. Bulmer, J. Lewis and D. Piachaud (eds), *The Goals of Social Policy*, London, Unwin Hyman.

Mullender, A. (1990) 'Employment-Related Day Care Needs in Nottingham', Nottingham, University of Nottingham Department of Social Work, unpublished.

Mullender, A. and Ward, D. (1988) 'What is Practice-led Research into Groupwork?', in P. Wedge (ed.), *Social Work – A Third Look at Research into Practice, Proceedings of the Third Annual JUC/BASW Conference*, held in London, September 1987, Birmingham, BASW.

Mullender, A. and Ward, D. (1989) 'Challenging Familiar Assumptions: preparing for and initiating a self-directed group', *Groupwork* 2 (1), 5–26.

Mullender, A. and Ward, D. (1991) *Self-Directed Groupwork: users take action for empowerment*, London, Whiting and Birch.

National Community Development Project (1973) *Inter-Project Report*, London, CDP Information and Intelligence Unit.

Network of Labour Community Research and Resources Centres, (1982) 'Pooling Our Resources', in G. Craig, N. Derricourt and M. Loney (eds), *Community Work and The State*, London, Routledge & Kegan Paul.

Nicolaus, M. (1972) 'Sociology Liberation Movement, a speech made to the 1968 convention of the American Sociological Association', in T. Pateman (ed.), *Counter Course: A Handbook for Course Criticism*, Harmondsworth, Penguin.

Nielsen, J. M. (ed.) (1990) *Feminist Research Methods: Exemplary Readings in the Social Sciences*, Boulder, Colorado, Westview Press.

Oakley, A. (1980) *Women Confined: Towards a Sociology of Childbirth*, Oxford, Martin Robertson.

Oakley, A. (1981) 'Interviewing Women: A contradiction in terms', in H. Roberts (ed.), *Doing Feminist Research*, London, Routledge & Kegan Paul.

O'Hagan, M. (1986) *From Taking Snap Shots to Making Movies: My Search for the Communication of Human Experience*, Auckland New Zealand, Mental Health Foundation.

Oliver, M. (1983) *Social Work with Disabled People*, London and Basingstoke, Macmillan.

Oliver, M. (1989) 'The social model of disability: current reflections', in P. Carter, T. Jeffs and M. Smith (eds), *Social Work and Social Welfare Yearbook 1*, Milton Keynes, Open University Press.

Parlett, M. and Hamilton, D. (1976) 'Evaluation as illumination: a new approach to the study of innovatory programmes', in D. A. Tawney (ed.), *Curriculum Evaluation Today: Trends and Implications*, Basingstoke, Macmillan.

Payne, M. (1991) *Modern Social Work Theory: a critical introduction*, Basingstoke, Macmillan.

Pearson, G., Treseder, J. and Yelloly, M. (eds) (1988) *Social Work and the Legacy of Freud: Psychoanalysis and its Uses*, Basingstoke, Macmillan Education.

Pease, R. (1990) 'Towards Collaborative Research on Socialist Theory & Practice in Social Work', in J. Petruchenia and R. Thorpe (eds), *Social Change and Social Welfare Practice*, Sydney, Hale and Iremonger.

Philip, A. E., McCulloch, J. W. and Smith, N. J. (1975) *Social Work Research and the Analysis of Social Data*, Oxford, Pergamon.

Pilcher, D.M. (1990) *Data Analysis for the Helping Professions: a practical guide*, London, Sage.

Pinker, R. (1978) *Research Priorities in the Personal Social Services*, Report to the Social Science Research Council, London.

Pinker, R. (1989) 'Social work and social policy in the twentieth century: retrospect and prospect', in M. Bulmer, J. Lewis and D. Piachaud (eds), *The Goals of Social Policy*, London, Unwin Hyman.

Platt, J. (1981) 'The social construction of 'positivism', and its significance in British sociology', in P. Abrams, R. Deem, J. Finch and P. Rock (eds), *Practice and Progress: British Sociology 1950–1980*, London, George Allen & Unwin.

Rafferty, E. (1991) 'Educational Affairs', *Social Work Today*, 20 June.

Reason, P. and Rowan, J. (eds) (1981) *Human Inquiry: A Sourcebook of New Paradigm Research*, Chichester, John Wiley and Sons.

Reid, W.J. and Shyne, A.W. (1969) *Brief and Extended Casework*, New York, Columbia University Press.

Reinharz, S. (1983) 'Experiential analysis: a contribution to feminist research', in G. Bowles and R. Duelli Klein (eds), *Theories of Women's Studies*, London, Routledge & Kegan Paul.

Richardson, S. (1989) 'Child sexual abuse: the challenge for the organization', in P. Carter, T. Jeffs and M. Smith *Social Work and Social Welfare Yearbook 1*, Milton Keynes, Open University Press.

Roberts, H. (ed.) (1981) *Doing Feminist Research*, London, Routledge & Kegan Paul.

Roberts, R. (1990) *Lessons from the Past: Issues For Social Work Theory*, London, Tavistock/Routledge.

Rogers, C.R. (1967) *On Becoming a Person: A Therapist's View on Psychotherapy*, London, Constable.

Rojek, C., Peacock, G. and Collins, S. (1988) *Social Work and Received Ideas*, London, Routledge.

Sainsbury, E. (1985) 'The Contribution of Client Studies to Social Work Practice', *Social Work – Research into Practice, Proceedings of the First Annual JUC/BASW Conference*, September 1985, London.

Sainsbury, E. (1987) 'Client Studies: their contribution and limitations in influencing social work practice', *British Journal of Social Work*, 17, (6), 635–644.

Sainsbury, E., Nixon, S. and Phillips, D., (1982) *Social Work in Focus: Clients', and Social Workers', Perceptions in Long-Term Social Work*, London, Routledge & Kegan Paul.

Scheffler, I. (1982) *Science and Subjectivity*, Indianapolis, Hackett.

Schon, D.A. (1983) *The Reflective Practitioner: how professionals think in action*, London, Temple Smith.

Seebohm Report (1968) *Report of the Committee on Local Authority and Allied Personal Social Services*, London, HMSO.

Shaw, I. (1975) 'Making use of research', in H. Jones (ed.), *Towards a New Social Work*, London, Routledge & Kegan Paul.

Shipman, M. (1988) *The Limitations of Social Research*, third edition, Harlow, Longman.

Silverman, D. (1985) *Qualitative Methodology and Sociology: Describing The Social World*, Aldershot, Gower.

Sims, D. (1981) 'From ethogeny to endogeny: how participants in research projects can end up doing research on their own awareness', in P. Reason and J. Rowan (eds), *Human Inquiry: A Sourcebook of New Paradigm Research*, Chichester, John Wiley and Sons.

Sinfield, A. (1969) *Which Way for Social Work?*, Fabian Tract 393, London, Fabian Society.

Smale, G. M. and Statham, D. (1989) 'Research into Practice: Using Research in Practice and Policy Making', in M. Stein (ed.), *Research into Practice: Proceedings of the Fourth Annual JUC/BASW Conference*, held at Leeds University, September 1988, Birmingham, BASW.

Smart, C. (1988) 'Researching Prostitution: Some Problems for Feminist Research', in Nebraska Sociological Feminist Collective, *A Feminist Ethic for Social Science Research*, Lewiston NY, Edwin Mellen Press.

Smith, B. and Noble-Spruell, C. (1986) 'An overview of feminist research perspectives', in H. Marchant and B. Wearing (eds), *Gender Reclaimed: Women in Social Work*, Sydney, Hale & Iremonger.

Smith, G. and Harris, R. (1972) 'Ideologies of need and the organisation of social work departments', *British Journal of Social Work*, 2(1).

Smith, M. (1988) *Developing Youth Work: informal education, mutual aid and popular practice*, Milton Keynes, Open University Press.

Spender, D. (1980) *Man Made Language*, London, Routledge & Kegan Paul.

Stanley, L. and Wise, S. (1983) *Breaking Out: Feminist Consciousness and Feminist Research*, London and New York, Routledge & Kegan Paul.

Stein, M. and Carey, K. (1986) *Leaving Care*, Oxford, Blackwell.

Taylor, I., Walton, P. and Young, J. (1973) *The New Criminology: For a social theory of deviance*, London, Routledge & Kegan Paul.

Taylor, I., Walton, P. and Young, J. (1975) *Critical Criminology*, London, Routledge & Kegan Paul.

Townsend, P. and Davidson, N. (eds) (1982) *The Black Report* London, Penguin.

Townsend, P., Phillimore, P. and Beattie, A. (1988) *Health and Deprivation: Inequality and the North*, London, Croom Helm.

Utting, W. (1989) 'Foreword' to B. Kahan (ed.), *Child Care Research, Policy and Practice*, London, Hodder & Stoughton.

Vernon, S., Harris, R. and Ball, C. (1990) *Towards Social Work Law: legally competent professional practice*, London, Central Council for Education and Training in Social Work.

Wadsworth, Y. (1982) 'The Politics of Social Research : a social research strategy for the community health, education and welfare movement', *Australian Journal of Social Issues*, 17 (3), 232–46.

Wadsworth, Y. (1984) *Do It Yourself Social Research*, Collingwood, Victoria, Victorian Council of Social Service and Melbourne Family Care Organisation in association with George Allen & Unwin.

Walby, S. (1990) *Theorizing Patriarchy*, Oxford, Blackwell.

Weedon, C. (1987) *Feminist Practice and Poststructuralist Theory*, Oxford, Blackwell.

Whitaker, D.S. and Archer, J.L. (1989) *Research by Social Workers: capitalizing on experience*, CCETSW Study 9, London, Central Council for Education and Training in Social Work.

Wilson, E. (1977) *Women and the Welfare State*, London, Tavistock.

Worrall, A. (1990) *Offending Women: Female Lawbreakers and the Criminal Justice System*, London, Routledge.

Yelloly, M.A. (1980) *Social Work Theory and Psychoanalysis*, London, Van Nostrand Reinhold.

Younghusband Report (1959) *Report of the Working Party on Social Workers in the Local Authority Health and Welfare Services*, London, HMSO.

Index of Authors

Index of Subjects